LLEWELL

2015
HERBAL
ALMANAC

© 2014 Llewellyn Publications is a registered
trademark of Llewellyn Worldwide Ltd.

Cover Design: Kevin R. Brown
Editing: Andrea Neff

Cover images:
iStockphoto.com/12008406,
10796750, 10711340, 10828080,
12001500, 11989058/Classix

Interior Art: © Fiona King

You can order annuals and books from
New Worlds, Llewellyn's catalog. To request
a free copy, call toll free: 1-877-NEW WRLD
or visit www.llewellyn.com.

ISBN 978-0-7387-2689-2
Llewellyn Worldwide Ltd.
2143 Wooddale Drive
Woodbury, MN 55125-2989

Printed in the United States of America

Contents

Herbs for Health and Beauty

Herb Crafts

Herb History, Myth, and Lore

Moon Signs, Phases, and Tables

Introduction to
Llewellyn's Herbal Almanac

More and more people are using herbs, growing and gathering them and studying them for their enlivening and healing properties. Whether in the form of a refreshing herbal tonic, a critter-friendly garden, or a new favorite recipe, herbs can clearly enhance your life.

In the 2015 edition of the *Herbal Almanac*, we once again feature some of the most innovative and original thinkers and writers on herbs. We tap into practical, historical, and just plain enjoyable aspects of herbal knowledge—using herbs to help you reconnect with the earth, enhance your culinary creations, and heal your body and mind. The thirty articles in this almanac will teach you everything from how to craft your own herbal tea blends to how to grow a window herb garden. You'll also learn how to create floral arrangements with herbs and flowers from your own garden, save seeds to share with family and friends, and improve your health with herbal remedies from your kitchen pharmacy. Enjoy!

Note: The old-fashioned remedies in this book are historical references used for teaching purposes only. The recipes are not for commercial use or profit. The contents are not meant to diagnose, treat, prescribe, or substitute consultation with a licensed health-care professional. Herbs, whether used internally or externally, should be introduced in small amounts to allow the body to adjust and to detect possible allergies. Please consult a standard reference source or an expert herbalist to learn more about the possible effects of certain herbs. You must take care not to replace regular medical treatment with the use of herbs. Herbal treatment is intended primarily to complement modern health care. Always seek professional help if you suffer from illness. Also, take care to read all warning labels before taking any herbs or starting on an extended herbal regimen. Always consult medical and herbal professionals before beginning any sort of medical treatment—this is particularly true for pregnant women. Herbs are powerful things; be sure you are using that power to achieve balance.

Llewellyn Worldwide does not participate in, endorse, or have any authority or responsibility concerning private business transactions between its authors and the public.

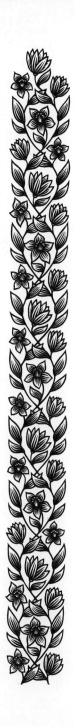

Growing
and
Gathering
Herbs

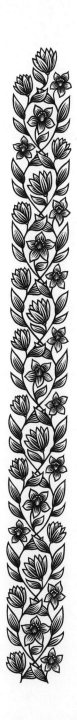

Seed Saving...Pass It On

⫸ By Monica Crosson ⫷

When I was first married, my husband and I bought a tiny cottage that I was determined to surround with the ideal fairytale garden.

Being young and having little money to buy planting material, I relied on the kindness of family and friends to share from their own gardens. My mother provided me with the bulk of my treasures, her own garden rivaling any in England. Soon my yard was teeming with daylilies, columbine, hollyhock, and iris from my mother, cuttings from my grandmother's heirloom roses, and starts from close friends. I loved and appreciated those plants that became part

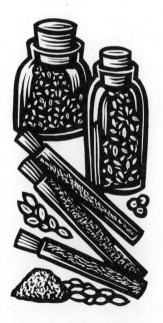

of my first garden. In fact, I called it my "story garden" because of the tales that were attached to each and every plant.

But one bright May morning, an unexpected visit by my in-laws started me down a gardening path shared by our ancestors but almost forgotten in recent times: seed saving.

My mother-in-law handed me a small glass baby food jar, and in the bottom was a scattering of silvery seeds.

I shook the jar a bit. "These look cool. What kind of seeds are these?"

"Well," she said sheepishly, "I don't know if they're any good, but they're honesty seeds. They were my grandmother's. I've had them in storage for a very long time, but I would like you to have them."

Honesty, also known as money plant or moonwort (*Lunaria annua*), is a biennial belonging to the Brassicaceae family. In its first year, the plant displays showy green leaves, but in the second year, it is covered with a riot of bright pink flowers. The mature seedpods resemble papery coins and are used in dried flower arrangements.

The next day, I scattered my little treasures under a southern-facing window. I watered them and watched patiently for three weeks for signs of life. Nothing.

Believing the seeds were no longer viable, I decided to plant English lavender there instead. But just before my shovel hit the dirt, I saw the lovely green shoots of the honesty plant pushing through the ground. The plants not only grew, they thrived. By their second season, they had grown to an astonishing six and a half feet tall and were covered with bright pink flowers.

That fall, I carefully collected the lovely silver moon-shaped seedpods and gave them away as thank-you tokens to all who had helped make my garden a success. That was twenty years ago, and I've been collecting and sharing seeds ever since.

Saving seeds can be as easy as shaking mature seed heads into containers at the end of their growing season. But there are other types of seed that require a bit more finesse. With a little knowledge and know-how, anyone can be a seed saver.

A Little History

For thousands of years, people saved seeds from the largest or most vigorous plants and replanted them, and then passed those seeds down from one generation to the next. This process created cultivars that were adapted to their region's growing conditions, which guaranteed flavor and made them naturally pest-resistant. In fact, as late as 1900 there were over 1,500 varieties of food crops, each further represented by thousands of different cultivated crops providing the world with food.

By the beginning of the twentieth century, farmers began to rely on seed companies, and soon the slower-selling seeds were dropped. This loss meant fewer seed choices and translated into lower genetic variability in our food plants. Loss of genetic seed diversity can lead to crop catastrophes. The Irish potato famine is an extreme example of what can happen when farmers rely on only a few plant species as their crop cornerstones. As we know, the Irish potato famine led to the death or displacement of two and a half million people in the 1840s.

Now there are fewer than thirty varieties of seed, and the top four (wheat, rice, corn, and soy) supply 75 percent of the calories we consume. Each time a seed variety is lost, we lose another chance to feed ourselves in a world of rising population and shrinking resources.

Why Save Seed

I began saving seed out of sentimentality, which is a great reason. Many heirloom varieties are threatened or extinct. Passing precious seed to family and friends not only preserves a bit of family history, but also preserves the genetic diversity of our heirloom food and flowering plants.

Saving seed also saves you money. I don't know about you, but it's really hard for me to pass up those brightly decorated seed packages, and at two to three dollars a packet, it adds up fast. It's not unusual for the average gardener to spend thirty to fifty dollars a year on seeds. Saving your own is free and keeps you away from those enticing seed displays. You can also trade seed with other seed savers in your neighborhood or join a seed exchange.

Most home gardeners don't realize that by saving their own seed from their largest plants, they can actually create new varieties that are adapted to their growing conditions. Doing this helps you maintain control of your own personal breeding goals.

Most commercial seeds are bred to improve shipping quality and the ability to be stored for long periods of time. The lower genetic variability of commercial seeds leads to lower adaptability to stresses such as pests or disease. Saving your own seed results in strong plants that are more resistant to pests and diseases in your region.

Terms to Know

Before you set off down the wonderful, rewarding path of seed saving, it's important to know a few basic terms.

Seeds

Seeds are living, hibernating plant embryos. They survive longest if kept in a cool, dark, dry place. Most plant seeds are viable for only a couple of years, but in some cases (such as my honesty plant) they can last longer.

Hybrids

Hybrids, also known as F1 hybrids, are plant varieties resulting from pollination between genetically distinct plants. Hybrid seeds may produce plants that die or yield few or no seeds, or they may not produce the same type of plants. Using hybrid seeds is definitely a no-no.

Heirlooms

These are plant varieties that have been nurtured, selected, and handed down for many generations. Some sources say that in order to be considered an heirloom, the variety must be at least one hundred years old. Others say fifty years old, and still others use the end of World War II (1945) as the starting point. There is still a lot of debate over this.

Annuals

An annual lives or grows for only one season. Annual flowers give one season of color to a garden. Most vegetables are annuals, too, growing and being harvested in one season. Annual seeds can be the easiest to collect.

Perennials

These are plants that live for at least two seasons. Perennials grow and bloom over the spring and summer and die back in the fall or winter. In the spring, they return again from their root stock.

Biennials

These are plants that require two years to complete their life cycle. During the first season, the plant remains compact and leafy. During the second season, flowering and seed formation occur, followed by the entire plant's death.

Pollination

This is the process of sexual fertilization in plants.

Open-Pollinated Plants

Open-pollinated plants (OPs) are stable plant varieties resulting from the pollination between the same or genetically similar parents. These plants are great for seed saving.

Self-Pollination

This type of pollination occurs without the need for other plants or flowers, because it takes place within the flower before it opens.

Cross-Pollination

This type of pollination takes place when pollen is exchanged between different flowers on the same or different plants.

Seed-Saving Techniques

Seed saving is fun and relatively easy, but here are a few tips that may help you avoid frustration.

First of all, hybrid varieties (look for the word "hybrid" or "F1 hybrid" in the description on the seed packet) do not always breed true to type. Avoid them. The easiest seeds to save are open-pollinating, non-hybrid annuals.

Many common vegetables (such as cabbages, root vegetables, Brussels sprouts, and parsley) are biennials and won't go to seed until their second year. In some regions, it may not even be possible to save seeds from certain biennial plants.

Finally, you can minimize the cross-fertilization process by planting only one variety of corn (or squash, tomato, etc.) at a time. Okay, let's get planting!

Vegetable and Fruit Seeds

I have always thought it best to start out simply. Here are some of the easiest vegetable and fruit seeds to save. Collect seeds from the fully mature, ripe fruit of these plants.

Beans, Peas, and Other Legumes

These are fun and the easiest of all. After you have enjoyed your bounty, pick a few plants on which to leave pods until they are "rattle dry." Pick the pods and remove the seeds when completely dry. If needed, you can pull entire plants after they have died down and hang them upside down in a garage or shed to finish the drying process.

Peppers

Select a mature pepper, preferably one that is completely red. It is recommended that you pick your pepper from the largest, most vigorous plant. Cut the pepper open, scrape the seeds onto a plate, and let the seeds dry in a non-humid, shaded place, testing them occasionally until they break rather than bend. Leave at room temperature until completely dry.

Pumpkins and Squash

Pumpkins and squash are at the seed-saving stage when you cannot dent them with a fingernail. Cut the plant open, scrape the seeds into a bowl, then wash, drain, and dry them. Seeds are dry when they break and no longer bend.

Eggplant

Leave the eggplant on the vine until it is yellow and hard. Remember to pick an eggplant from your largest, most vigorous plant. Cut the eggplant in half and pull the flesh away from the seeded area. Dry the seeds on a plate for one to two weeks.

Cucumbers

Cucumbers turn yellow after they ripen and start to become mushy. Cut the cucumber in half and scrape the seeds into a bowl. You want to remove their slimy coating. You can do this by rubbing them gently around the inside of a sieve while washing them, or soak them in water for two days. Rinse and dry. Seeds are dry when they break and no longer bend.

Tomatoes

Tomatoes seeds are a little trickier because they are encased in a gelatinous coating, which prevents them from sprouting inside the tomato. You need to remove this coating by fermenting it. This basically mimics the natural rotting of the fruit and has the added bonus of killing seed-borne tomato disease. Squeeze the seeds from a fully ripe tomato into a bowl, then add water and let stand at room temperature for about three days. You will know fermentation has occurred because mold will form on the surface of the water. Add more water, stir, then gently scrape mold and debris off the top. Repeat until only clean seed remains, then strain, rinse, and leave the seeds at room temperature until they are thoroughly dry—about one to two weeks.

Flower Seeds

The first seeds I saved were from heirloom flowers, and they're still my favorite. I mostly choose annual and perennial plants that are known for keeping their characteristics each generation. Instead of pinching off all of the spent flowers after they have bloomed, let a few develop seedpods. When the seeds are dry, shake them into a bag. It's that easy! Here are some of my favorites to save.

Foxglove

Foxglove *(Digitalis purpurea)* is a biennial plant with soft, hairy, toothed, ovate leaves in a basal rosette. Its trumpet-like blossoms are beautiful but very poisonous.

Hollyhock

Hollyhock *(Alcea rosea)* is a biennial that grows up to ten feet tall, with broad, rounded, lobed leaves and numerous flowers on the erect central stem.

Nasturtium

Nasturtium *(Tropaeolum majus)* is an annual with edible peppery-tasting leaves that are sometimes used in salads. The brilliant yellow, orange, or red flowers are funnel-shaped, with a long spur.

Sweet Pea

The strong-growing vines of the sweet pea *(Lathyrus odoratus)* bear a profusion of colorful 1 ½-inch flowers in the typical form of the pea family. This is an old-fashioned favorite.

Beebalm

Beebalm *(Monarda didyma)*, a perennial with its distinctive square stem, is a member of the mint family. It grows two to three feet tall and has red, purple, or pink crown-like flowers that smell amazing.

Storing Seeds

When storing your seeds, you need to think dry and cool. Humidity and warmth shorten a seed's shelf life. I keep my seeds in paper envelopes tucked into labeled Mason jars in the pantry on the main floor of my house. Your refrigerator is also a good choice. Be sure to label your container with the variety, the date, and other pertinent information, and try to avoid opening the container until you are ready to plant.

Stored seeds will retain their viability for different lengths of time depending on the type of seed. Most seed is good for about two years.

Making a Difference

There are many organizations out there that are dedicated to the revival of seed saving and exchange. The most well-known one is Seed Savers Exchange, a nonprofit organization dedicated to saving and sharing heirloom seeds. They have a wonderful catalog with an amazing array of seeds.

An organization near and dear to my heart is Finney Farm. They grow and collect seed from a variety of heirloom and open-pollinated vegetables. Instead of marketing their wares as a source of income, they give them away to food banks, at fairs and markets, and to anyone who requests them. Their goal is to have more people grow their own food, preserve heirloom varieties, and encourage species diversity for the health of the planet and people.

You can make a difference, too. Once you have a nice selection of seeds and/or heirloom plant starts, host an exchange party. Invite friends, family, and neighbors to bring plant starts or seeds to share. After snacking and sharing stories about your treasures, let everyone take as many as they brought. If you don't know anyone who gardens, pique your friends' interest by giving them a packet of your very own seeds, a terracotta pot, and a small bag of potting soil. Give your seeds to a local food bank or pass them out at a farmers' market.

Feel satisfied and more connected to the earth by cultivating and sharing seeds, and empower yourself with the knowledge that you are in control of what you grow and feed your family.

It's been a long time since those first tiny seeds captured my heart. We grew to a family of five and sold the cottage. We built another house just across the river from where I planted that first garden. I took with me plenty of starts and jars full of seeds. Now, when I look out across my lawn, I still see daylilies, columbine, hollyhock, and iris originating from my mother's garden, cuttings from my grandmother's heirloom roses, as well as those wonderful starts from close friends. I still have honesty plants that grow in my border, too. And when my children get older and have gardens of their own, I will pass on to them the precious gift of a seed.

Resources

Ashworth, Suzanne. *Seed to Seed*. Decorah, IA: Seed Savers Exchange, 1991.

Finney Farm. "Seed Distro Project." www.finneyfarm.org /Seed_Distro.html.

Seed Savers Exchange. www.seedsavers.org.

Monica Crosson *is a Master Gardener who lives in the beautiful Pacific Northwest, happily digging in the dirt and tending her raspberries with her husband, three kids, two goats, two dogs, three cats, a dozen chickens, and Rosetta the donkey. She is the author of* Summer Sage, *a novel for tweens. Visit her at www.monicacrosson.com.*

So You Want to Grow a Window Herb Garden

By Tess Whitehurst

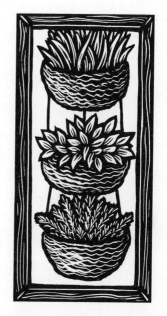

Doesn't every herb enthusiast want fresh herbs at their fingertips year round? For this purpose, live indoor herbs are the way to go—and they're fairly simple to grow. Not only that, but they look lovely and add such a homegrown coziness to any kitchen décor. So whether you're a rookie or an old hat at indoor herb gardening, read on for a mishmash of practical and unique tips for establishing and maintaining your very own fragrant, medicinal, culinary, and attractive indoor garden of delights.

Choosing Your Herbs

Herbs that grow well indoors include basil, catnip, chervil, chives, coriander,

lemon balm, mint, oregano, parsley, rosemary, sage, savory, tarragon, and thyme.

Location, Location, Location

If you're just starting out, you'll want to choose a windowsill,
greenhouse window, or glass shelf in a recessed window that
gets a lot of sun throughout the day. Six hours of direct sunlight are ideal for most herbs, although there are some variations from herb to herb, so be sure to keep this in mind when
choosing your herbs and your location.

In some cases and during the darker time of the year, you
may want to place a fluorescent or grow light near your herbs
to help them get the required amount of light.

It's important to note that although herbs enjoy very good
soil drainage, most of them also enjoy balmy air. For this reason, if you live in a dry climate, it can be a good idea to place
them over the kitchen sink if possible, so that they can benefit
from the rising steam. Regularly misting your herbs with water
is another way to help them meet their humidity requirements.

Unique Display Ideas

If you don't have a flat surface to spare, or if you just love the
novelty of it, you might want to hang your herbs. There are a
number of fun ways to do this. For example, once you locate
an appropriate sunny window, you might:

- Place your herb pots in hanging buckets and attach them
  with hooks or clothespins to a suspended curtain rod.

- Line a three-tiered metal hanging basket with peat moss.
  Fill the rest with soil, and plant herbs in each basket.

- Look around at various hanging planters specifically
  designed for indoor herbs. There are a number on the

market these days, so take your time and find one or two that you like.

- Plant your herbs in coffee cans, and hang them upside down. (There are a number of blogs with detailed instructions on how to do this.)

Additionally, there are plenty of other fun and crafty ways to display your herbs. For example, you may choose to plant your herbs in attractive antique tins, antique teapots, tea tins, or coffee cans. Just pierce drainage holes at the bottom, line them with gravel, and place them on top of a saucer or long tray (to catch excess water).

Planting

If you're an experienced gardener, go ahead and grow your herbs from seeds if you so desire. But if you're not as confident with the color of your thumb, just go with the starters! They're so much easier and they're very reasonably priced.

Good soil drainage is of the essence, so it can be a good idea to choose unglazed clay pots and consider adding a bit of gravel or broken terracotta pot shards to the bottom. Smaller pots (five-inch pots or so) are fine for most herbs, but basil likes a larger pot to accommodate its larger root system.

Watering and Feeding

Water your herbs thoroughly and regularly. A good rule of thumb is to water them enough so that some water drains out of the bottom, and then to give them enough time to dry out before their next watering (but not too much time). You could start by watering once every day or two, and then adjust this as needed for each plant. You might find that your plants' water requirements vary throughout the year, depending on the duration of sunlight and degree of heat, so regulate accordingly. If you grow basil, the appearance of its leaves can be a good litmus test for whether or not your herbs have enough water, so a little trick is to keep an eye on the basil.

When it comes to feeding, herbs generally grow to be more flavorful when they are not in overly rich soil, so in most cases you won't want to over-fertilize. And when you do fertilize—perhaps once every one or two weeks—dissolve something gentle and natural into your watering can, such as weak coffee (one part weak coffee to four parts water) or a small amount of coffee grounds or seaweed fertilizer.

What to Do about Bugs

Even though many herbs naturally deter pests, sometimes bugs may still be attracted to your indoor garden. If this starts to be a problem, mix one teaspoon mild, eco-friendly dish soap with a gallon of tepid water. After protecting the base of the plant with a plastic bag or with your hand, spray the solution on the leaves and allow it to dry naturally. Make sure your plants are thoroughly coated (pay attention to the top and bottom of the leaves), but don't spray more than is necessary. Alternatively, if the leaves are broader, you might use the solution to wipe the leaves off using a sponge or paper towel, again paying attention to both the top and bottom of the leaves. Repeat this process every three days until your pest problem is no more.

Herb-Specific Growing and Harvesting Ideas

Although most herbs have generally similar care needs, each one is, of course, slightly different. So depending on the herbs you choose, you'll want to keep the following guidance in mind.

Because it's important to lightly harvest your herbs regularly by taking snips and clippings here and there (as this keeps your plants vibrant and healthy), I've included some unique (and some not-so-unique) ideas for employing your herbs, just in case you haven't been cooking lately or you're running out of recipe ideas. Just be sure to snip and pluck the more tender leaves from the top rather than the sturdier and more established leaves at the bottom, as this will ensure that your plant will fill out properly rather than getting spindly or top-heavy.

Basil likes a bit more sun than most other herbs, perhaps somewhere in the vicinity of eight hours a day rather than six. It also likes to stay fairly hot, ideally at 80 degrees or so. Basil also differs from many other window herbs in that it prefers a larger pot—perhaps twelve inches or larger—to accommodate its roots. Employ basil in a pinch (literally!) by putting fresh leaves in your salad, soup, and sandwiches or on top of your pizza. You can also dry the leaves and save them for later use.

Catnip's leaves grow most abundantly when you're diligent about pinching off flowers as soon as they appear. Make sure to keep the soil constantly moist. Employing catnip shouldn't be any trouble at all to those with catnip-loving cats. (Reportedly, not all cats feel the buzz, and kittens usually don't until they're at least six months to a year old.) Pinch off fresh leaves for your cat to enjoy, or dry the leaves, then put them in cat toys or sprinkle over cat treats. Catnip tea, for humans, can help soothe the stomach and calm the nerves.

Chives like bright light; six to eight hours is best. Again, just dry if you can't seem to find enough uses for the fresh herb.

Coriander is another herb that likes a little more sun—six to eight hours a day rather than just six. You can add fresh coriander leaves to Mexican or Asian dishes, salsas, and dips or to soups and salads. You can also use this herb when you get takeout, heat up a frozen dinner, or throw together a burrito for lunch. Coriander tea soothes stomach cramps and reduces bloating. Oh, and blend the fresh leaves into a mango and cilantro margarita—yum!

Lemon balm doesn't need as much sun as your average indoor herb; at least four hours a day should do the trick. Add dried lemon balm to medicinal teas used for soothing the stomach, reducing menstrual cramps, and calming the nerves. Fresh, crushed lemon balm can be a delicious and unique addition to refreshing cocktails and beverages.

Mint comes in a huge number of varieties, so take your time and choose the one(s) you really want. It's best for mint to receive primarily morning sunlight, as it can scorch in hotter temperatures. As with basil, be sure to pinch off the flowering tops when they appear to ensure plentiful leaves. Fresh mint leaves add refreshing coolness to bathwater. Mint is also great for mojitos and other cold cocktails—try it in a blended margarita! And just a sprig in iced tea or lemonade is a simple, gourmet finishing touch. Add dried mint to herbal tea blends for flavor and to lift the spirits, clear the mind, and soothe the stomach.

Oregano can thrive after spending a few weeks outdoors when the weather is warm. When it's indoors, be sure to rotate it every now and then so it receives light evenly. Add oregano to your pesto recipes, chop it and sprinkle over frozen or homemade pizzas before baking, or—the old standby—dry it and save it for later.

Parsley likes to go a little gentler on the light: four to six hours a day rather than the standard six. Also, it likes to stay in cooler temperatures, around 65 to 70 degrees. Fresh parsley adds a super-healthy blast of deliciousness to green smoothies. For example, try throwing it in the blender with spinach, an apple, coconut water, fresh ginger, and frozen pineapples and/or frozen red grapes. Of course, it's also a great last-minute addition to salads, soups, sandwiches, and any number of savory dishes.

Rosemary is quite a hardy little plant, so you might want to choose rosemary if you're a beginner at indoor herb gardening. Just be sure that your plant gets plenty of light, and allow the soil to dry between waterings. To enhance memory, clarity, and focus, rub a sprig of rosemary between your fingers to release the scent, and then inhale. The flavor and health benefits of many a store-bought soup can be enhanced by grinding a few leaves of rosemary thoroughly with a mortar and pestle and then adding them to the pot.

Sage prefers to stay moist, but be sure to drain any excess water out of its saucer so its roots don't get soggy. Also, rinse the leaves every month or two to keep them dust-free. Dry sage and safely burn the leaves as you would incense, to impart a fresh, smoky scent to your home. Sage tea can help with menopause and night sweats.

Savory is particularly easy to grow. Just be extra certain that the soil has time to drain and dry out between waterings. Add savory to soups, salads, rice dishes, pastas, and steamed vegetables.

Tarragon, like basil, likes a deeper pot for its root system, so find a pot that's at least twelve inches deep. Add tarragon to soups and salads, or dry it and use for tea to soothe digestion and relax the body and nervous system.

Thyme is drought-resistant, so while you want to water it regularly, you also want to make doubly sure that it gets plenty of time to dry out between waterings. This herb isn't known for its longevity, so if your thyme's life cycle seems to be on the wane, just eat as much thyme as you can before it's gone, and then replace it. Dried thyme can be incorporated into tea blends to help heal colds and support immunity.

A Lifelong Friendship

Having and tending a window herb garden can be a beautifully symbiotic, lifelong friendship: you care for the herbs, and they care for you. Enjoy the process! Experiment with what works best in your home, get in the habit of incorporating fresh herbs into your dietary and health regimens, and enhance all the days of your life with these delicious, delightful little beings.

Tess Whitehurst *is an intuitive counselor, energy worker, feng shui consultant, and author of* Magical Housekeeping, The Good Energy Book, The Art of Bliss, The Magic of Flowers, *and* Magical Fashionista. *She has appeared on the Bravo TV show* Flipping Out, *and her writing has been featured in* Writer's Digest *and online at* Whole Life Times Magazine *and* AOL/Huffington Post. *She lives in Venice, CA. Visit her online (and discover her blogs and free monthly newsletter) at tesswhitehurst.com.*

Critter-Friendly Gardening: Keeping Your Garden Safe for All

≫ By Diana Rajchel ≪

Bunnies are cute. Raccoons are clever. Bugs are, like it or not, a necessity. Add your garden to their environment and all of the above can become a nuisance. You may think of that garden as your territory, but the other creatures of the earth just don't recognize property rights. To grow with abundance, you must lay down boundaries that animals understand.

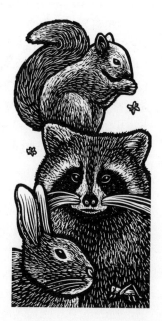

Some people like to trap and re-lease their pestiferous critters, but this can take a lot more time and energy than a gardener with a day job might have. Rather than expend your energy in street wars with squirrels, you can cultivate a garden that critters choose not to visit.

Establish Borders

The simplest way to keep curious critters away from your garden is to erect a barrier. Chicken wire around a plot is cheap and effective. Some gardeners, however, bemoan the way the chicken wire looks, and moving it to do your gardening work is a hassle. Also, it's not absolutely effective against larger animals. An occasional intrepid rabbit can find its way between the slots, leading it to paroxysms of joy as it consumes your entire lettuce patch. While decorative fences might tempt you, save those for guiding human visitors down garden paths. A one-foot-tall white plastic fence means nothing to rabbits or gophers.

If you do not want to fence your entire garden, just focus on specific plants. You can net plants individually, perhaps leaving one or two for the wilderness.

Raised garden beds also reduce animal interest in your garden. By elevating it slightly above the ground, you can keep a close eye on what may lurk between your rows (or circles). Raised beds also keep out slugs and other animals that can't climb. However, for anything that flies or tunnels, the garden remains fair game.

You can keep out most slugs by cutting a one-liter plastic bottle in half (leaving roughly six to ten inches) and placing it over the plant with the open bottle at the top. If this offends you aesthetically, you may prefer to embed a small amount of copper wire around your plants. It creates a miniature electric fence—not enough to shock a human-size creature but enough to put off slugs.

If electrocution seems too cruel, go with a little necessary roughness. Pieces of granite or sandpaper littered throughout the garden paths can deter the most intrepid of wandering critters. Some gardeners prefer to use coffee grounds for texture.

If you grow grapes, you especially need to watch out for bees and birds. Place paper bags over the bunches as they appear. This protects grapes from diseases and vine-withering stingers. This also makes sure that the birds don't eat all of them. The leaves on the plant are what require exposure to light, so as long as you leave them uncovered, the rest of the fruit can ripen inside the paper bag.

Choose Repellent Plants

Companion planting is a theory of gardening that suggests that certain plants grow better in close proximity to one another. It can also be used as a means of environmentally safe pest control. For example, as one plant drains the soil of nitrogen, the other may resupply it. If your basil attracts a lot of Japanese beetles, you might slow them down by planting something they hate between the basil plants. Pretend your garden is actually a small community of plant people (perhaps a Doomsday cult, since you will eventually eat most of them). Each plant you install has a specific role in service to its community.

When you share a garden, companion planting becomes especially important. When my neighbors informed me that our collective backyard serves as both garden and rabbit sanctuary, my pest control choices narrowed. After all, there could be no rabbit casualties. Thus the first plant seeded was marigolds. Pests of all kinds from rabbits to bugs hate marigolds. So the outer edge of my garden is now a bright orange.

Still, marigolds alone did not seem like enough to keep away the determined bunny or adventurous squirrel. However, adaptation has made bugs far more persistent and frustrating when it comes to gardening. So I added plants that have evolved a "don't eat me" gene: peppers. I then planted onions as close as possible to my protected crops of onions and green beans.

It amused me to watch the insect reaction to peppers: every so often, I would see a single bite on a pepper leaf. That was usually all the insect wanted before moving on to greener snacks.

Certain plants repel certain bugs more than others, and other plants might do great things for your garden but awful things for your pets.

The following list can help you determine what to add as deterrents to keep the pests away from your hard work.

Aphids
Deterrents: Onions, garlic, leeks, chervil, cilantro, dill, fennel, oregano, sunflower.

California Beetles
Deterrents: Beans (all kinds).

Pests of All Kinds
Deterrents: Mustard, parsnip, rhubarb.

Beetles
Deterrents: Radishes, hemp, tansy, geraniums, lemon balm, marigolds, catnip.

Mosquitoes
Deterrents: Basil, southernwood, artemisias.

Flies
Deterrents: Cilantro, peppermint, basil.

In the Upper Midwest, the chief challenges come from aphids, Japanese beetles, wasps, and persistent rabbits, squirrels, and cats. The critters of concern for you may change completely depending on the region and sometimes just based on the adaptivity of the animals. For instance, in the past decade, Saint Paul, Minnesota, has seen an increase in bear visits. Gardeners may need to dig deep, because chicken wire and marigolds won't do much to stop an animal that size.

Don't just rely on one plant to act as a repellent. Bugs can develop resistance to natural chemicals (from plants) just as much as they can to synthetic sources. Slow this process by switching out crops every year (or few years). The variety keeps the bugs from winning and gives your soil a nice break once in a while.

Mix Up Animal-Safe Repellents

The miracle household chemical of the twentieth century is still amazing today: dish soap. It is the single most effective tool available for keeping the critters from chomping your harvest, but it also has some serious drawbacks when it comes to its long-term impact on the whole ecosystem beyond just your own garden.

Overuse can leave too much salt in your soil and risks poisoning the groundwater and ultimately throwing off the algae balance of any nearby natural water supply. You can get around this concern by using a phosphate-free detergent. Unfortunately, phosphate-free does not automatically mean its safe for your environment. Fragrances, dyes, and other cleaning agents may impact the soil in ways that we haven't had a chance to see yet. If you do use this—and in some cases the only way to save a garden is to trot out the machine-made mix—use it as sparingly as possible and as diluted with water as the insect response will allow.

If you're in a well-balanced place with the bug population, it's likely a better long-term strategy to use other plants as a means to manage them. You can grow some of these directly as deterrent plants, or sprinkle peelings and leftover plant pieces throughout your garden. The following list can give you a general idea of what to use based on your animal challenge.

Rabbits
Deterrents: Onions, garlic, trace amounts of soap, hot peppers.

Cats
Deterrents: Sprinkle citrus peels throughout the garden, hot peppers.

Dogs
Deterrents: Citrus, vinegar (only on outer edges of garden—vinegar can kill plants), hot peppers.

Deer
Deterrents: Use a raw-egg base and mix with other hot things such as tabasco, onions, garlic, and hot pepper. Spray over the area that deer visit the most. The egg makes the formula stick for a long time.

Squirrels, Moles, and Gophers
Deterrents: Castor oil mixed with other deterrent plants or phosphate-free soap.

Insects
Deterrents: Thyme, onion, garlic, neem, tea tree oil, eucalyptus.

An all-purpose critter repellent might include a solution of citrus peel, garlic powder, cayenne powder, several peppers, a trace amount of vinegar, and essential oils. Several extreme cruelty-free and low-carbon-footprint gardeners also recommend urine, but most people find the prospect too gross to pursue.

Use a very light hand with repellent sprays—one spray right after each rainfall is really all you need. If you must use soap, nine parts water to one part soap is an optimal dilution. If you feel uncomfortable even risking this much soap use, use an equally dilute vinegar solution with extreme care. Vinegar can also be an herbicide, so save this for extreme measures.

Fertilize Safely

A common and much-decried practice among gardeners is the use of fertilizers created from decomposed animal flesh. The animal flesh, unfortunately, is also one way to send a very clear signal to animals that they don't want to tread there. Blood meal, for instance, is dried and powdered blood. It deters rabbits and enriches soil—but also feels much too morbid for the average animal lover. Some very effective alternatives involve decayed plants rather than decayed animals.

Mulch

You can use just about any light-blocking biodegradable material as mulch. While compost—the decayed leftovers of gardens and plant–based edibles past—is usually the popular mulch of choice, other methods can choke out weeds without harming any nearby animals. For example, after the first weeding of the season, lay down newspapers that effectively block out light to the weeds while leaving the plants you want to grow uncovered. Grass clippings and weeds also make great mulch covering. An up-and-coming mulch/fertilizer that might surprise you is seaweed. Not only does it keep weeds to minimum, but insects find seaweed gross and confusing, so they taste it once and leave the salad bar. So do all the other North American critters that do not generally encounter plants that originated in saltwater. Seaweed is also highly abundant and renewable, making it a great choice for mulch and fertilizer. If you live close to a coast, you can go gather the seaweed yourself. Otherwise, organic gardening shops do have it available in liquid form.

Infusions

Your plants do enjoy a nice cup of tea. A mixture of nettle, dandelion, and comfrey chopped and soaked in a bucket under the sun for a day gives them a nutritious refresher—and won't harm any of the animals in your area. You can also work some repellent plants into this mix: adding garlic or onion peels gives them a nice bit of insulation against encroaching animals.

Safe Plants

For those who simply want the bugs off but don't want pets or bunnies endangered, choose plants with care. For example, castor beans do a great job getting ride of moles but make dogs very ill. The risks to your pet might outweigh the benefits of losing the moles.

For an exhaustive list of possible garden dangers to your pet, please check the list available from the American Society for the Prevention of Cruelty to Animals, at www.aspca.org/pet-care/animal-poison-control/toxic-and-non-toxic-plants.

Common Garden Plants Dangerous to Dogs (and Cats, in Some Cases)

Azaleas, baby's breath, begonias, calla lily, cape jasmine, castor bean, chamomile, cyclamen, daffodils, dahlias, daisy, garlic, geranium, gladiola, grapes, hops, hyacinth, hydrangea, iris, lilies, walnuts.

Common Garden Plants Dangerous Only to Cats

Crocus, cherries, eucalyptus, lily of the valley, lobelia, milfoil, morning glory, narcissus, St. John's wort, tomato, tulips, wisteria, yarrow, yew.

Coexist

There are gardeners who prefer to share with the creatures around them. If bugs are especially enthused about a certain plant, you can plant one away from the rest of your garden just for them. You may prefer to trap and relocate certain animals. Just keep in mind that removing insects is a limited strategy: no matter how many you move, there are always more coming.

If you don't want to share your goodies with the neighborhood critters, the rules are the same as they are for human conduct: establish firm boundaries. Failing that, do what you can to drive them away. Be gentle—no need to lay waste to the land. Especially be gentle if you have pets or children in your care. A poison-free approach to gardening is better for everyone.

Diana Rajchel *lives and works in a Northeast Minneapolis townhouse. She shares this space with her life partner, at least two robots, and a warren of rabbits that her neighbors insist she tolerate.*

Because of said warren, she uses her gardening space to grow peppers and pungent herbs that rodents are loath to raid. Diana is also a journalist, author, poet, and occasional prankster. You can read more about her at http://blog.dianarajchel.com.

Fantastic Fennel

≫ By Jill Henderson ≪

Among the many wonderful herbs available to the gardener, no honest-to-goodness herb garden is truly complete without at least one tall, stately fennel plant. I say that because fennel is not only edible, medicinal, and downright gorgeous, but it also attracts hordes of beneficial insects and butterflies to the garden.

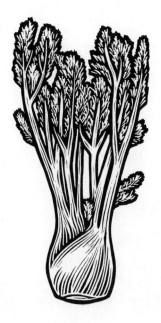

Despite its obvious charms, fennel is one of those herbs that even long-time gardeners seem to overlook. Indeed, I am always surprised by gardeners who mistake my fennel for dill. Perhaps it is the fern-like leaves or the umbels of bright yellow flowers—after all, the two are closely related and have a very similar shape and form. But once you have grown fennel in your own garden and tasted its luscious anise-like flavor, you will never mistake it for anything else.

Types of Fennel

Cultivated fennel comes in three basic varieties, all of which belong to the vast and diverse Apiaceae (parsley) family of plants. A few members of this family are common culinary herbs, such as parsley, dill, cilantro/coriander, anise, and fennel, as well as several traditional vegetables, including carrots, celery, and parsnips.

There are three varieties of cultivated fennel, including:

- Sweet fennel *(Foeniculum vulgare dulce)*

- Bronze fennel *(Foeniculum vulgare dulce* var. *'Rubrum' or 'Purpureum')*

- Florence fennel *(Foeniculum vulgare* var. *azoricum)*

All true fennels begin their first growing season as a basal rosette of finely dissected, fern-like leaves, which quickly grow into thick upright stalks that can reach upwards of five feet or more before flowering. Fennel leaves are finely dissected, with a swollen stem base that clasps the main stalk in a thin membrane. As the plant matures, new leaves and flowering umbels emerge from within the protection of these papery sheaths. Florence fennel does the same thing, only its leaf stems are thick and bulbous and grow so closely together that they form a nearly solid mass close to the ground.

The tiny, bright yellow flowers of fennel are born singly atop long, thin pedicels (tiny stems) that are bunched tightly together in clusters of twenty to fifty to form the classic flat-topped umbels so closely identified with members of the parsley family. Once the flowers begin to fade, elongated and slightly ribbed fruits emerge. As the fruits dry, they turn varying shades of brown, eventually splitting into two individual seeds.

The first seed heads of the season are known as "primaries." They are always the largest in diameter and produce the most and the largest seeds. Each successive wave produces seed heads that are just a bit smaller than the ones before.

As you might deduce from its Latin name, sweet fennel (*Foeniculum vulgare dulce*) is the original and classic form of this delightful herb. It is a tall, stately plant reaching heights of well over five feet when in bloom. Its seed are large, sweet, and richly aromatic.

When speaking of fennel as a medicinal herb, sweet fennel is the variety of choice. Not only does it outrank the other varieties by its size and productiveness, but its seeds contain the highest concentration of medicinally active volatile oils. It also has the strongest and, some say, the best flavor of them all.

Florence fennel (*Foeniculum vulgare* var. *azoricum*) is known as "finocchio" in Italy and is occasionally mislabeled as "anise" here in the United States. This fennel is known and grown around the world for its fleshy, celery-like lower stems, which grow so closely together as to create an oblong, slightly flattened, fan-shaped orb commonly referred to as a "bulb." Fennel bulbs are sweet, tender, and crispy, with a mild licorice or anise-like flavor.

Although Florence fennel is primarily cultivated as a vegetable, it will also produce flowers and set large, flavorful seeds, but only if the bulb goes unharvested.

Of the three fennel varieties, my all-time favorite is the absolutely lovely and always impressive bronze fennel (*Foeniculum vulgare dulce* var. 'Rubrum' or 'Purpureum'). While its seeds are quite small (often less than one-sixteenth of an inch long) and relatively mild in flavor when compared to the other varieties, I actually prefer them for cooking because they are unobtrusive when added to foods.

I also love the way bronze fennel works as a focal point in the garden. The stems are mostly green, with dashes of deep maroon or purple throughout. Early in the season, the leaves are dramatically colored, with a mixture of deep blue-green and bronze hues. Of course, one can't talk about bronze fennel without mentioning the literal profusion of delicate yellow flower umbels that light up this herb for weeks on end. This is a fennel that is more than pretty enough for the flower garden.

How Does Your Fennel Grow?

Sweet and bronze fennel are hardy perennials suitable for most climates, but they prefer long seasons of relatively warm, dry weather. Florence fennel is a little more demanding of water than the other two. While fennel plants can withstand a lot of abuse, they are not reliably perennial in areas that experience long periods of severe cold.

Growing fennel from seed is easy as long as you are using very fresh seed. Seeds stored for more than two years will likely not germinate.

Like other members of the parsley family, fennel has a long main taproot and does not transplant well. For this reason, it is best to sow fennel a quarter-inch deep directly in the garden. While seed can be planted in early spring, I prefer to sow seed in early to late winter. This method is known as "winter sowing" and has many advantages over traditional spring plantings, including earlier and stronger germination, seedlings that are well adapted to spring weather, and lack of transplant shock. Once the seeds are sown, they will germinate when weather conditions are exactly right for them.

After seedlings have reached eight to ten inches tall, they should be thinned to stand six inches apart, with a final spacing of twelve to fourteen inches for Florence fennel and twenty-four to thirty-six inches for seed-bearing varieties.

Like many other herbs, fennel needs little in the way of supplemental fertilizer to keep it growing strong. Even if growing fennel in average soil, a weekly watering and a light side-dressing of bone meal around seed fennels prior to flowering are all that is needed. When growing seed fennel, consider staking plants as the seed heads develop. For this, a light bamboo cage or trellis should do the trick.

While seed-bearing fennels are easy to care for, Florence fennel has a reputation for being fussy. It doesn't need extravagantly wonderful soil, but it will bolt on a dime if a cool spring suddenly turns hot or the plants are not provided with a steady supply of moisture. One way to prevent premature bolting is by keeping the soil temperature as steady as possible. This is easily accomplished by applying a one-inch layer of mulch when seedlings are about six inches tall and steadily increasing the depth as plants grow taller. Up to six inches of mulch applied early in the season will go a long way in keeping the soil cool and moist.

The mulch you apply in spring will also come in handy when the Florence fennel bulbs begin to mature. Simply pull enough mulch up and around the bulbs to block the sunlight from reaching them. Blanching keeps the bulbs light in color, crisp, and sweet. It also helps prevent dirt and grit from becoming entrenched in the tightly wrapped stems.

Fennel and Flying Flowers

Fennel and other herbs in the parsley family, such as anise, caraway, dill, and parsley, are all food hosts for swallowtail butterfly larvae. The female lays her eggs on the host plant, and the caterpillars emerge with an abundant supply of food at hand. If removed from their specific host plants, these caterpillars will die of starvation.

Keep in mind that a few caterpillars won't completely destroy a large host plant, but they do feed ravenously on both leaves and flower umbels, which can reduce yield and make plants look thin and straggly.

Because bronze fennel is a major focal point in my herb garden, I like to keep it looking as nice as possible. But I also hate the idea of killing the caterpillars, since I really enjoy having butterflies around all summer. So instead of killing the caterpillars, I plant extra fennel in another bed, along with other parsley family members and several flowering plants that the adult butterflies feed on. This way, when I find caterpillars munching on the fennel in the herb garden, I can simply move them to the butterfly garden, where they can continue their metamorphosis in peace.

A Little Fennel Goes a Long Way

Gardeners who practice companion planting are well aware that some plants don't like each other very much and will grow poorly if planted too close together. Fennel is one of those herbs that many garden crops (particularly bush beans, tomatoes, and onions) just don't like very much. That's because fennel is an allelopathic plant whose roots and leaves produce a biochemical that can inhibit the growth of other plants nearby. This compound literally reduces any competition from unrelated plants by clearing the way for fennel's own progeny. That being said, not all plants respond negatively to fennel. Indeed, the oregano, thyme, and French sorrel growing alongside the bronze fennel in my garden don't seem to mind it the least bit.

By now, you probably realize that fennel is a very hardy and self-determined herb. In addition to its ability to thwart the competition, it also produces a plethora of tiny seeds that are easily scattered near and far. Because of this, fennel can and will become invasive if the seed heads are allowed to mature on the plant and shatter. To help reduce the chances of this happening, all seed heads should be gathered before they ripen.

As soon as the first few seeds in each umbel turn brown, snip off the entire head with a pair of scissors and place in a large paper bag, where the seeds will continue to ripen and dry. Gather seed heads every few days until the entire harvest is complete. Once all of the seeds are brown and dry, they can be rolled between the palms to release them from their tiny stems.

It is often said that cilantro can be used to control the unwanted spread of fennel in the garden. While I haven't yet tried to prove or disprove this bit of garden lore, I can say with certainty that I've never had fennel growing in my cilantro.

For such a sturdy perennial, fennel is not oblivious to foul winter weather. In areas with very cold winters or repeated freeze-and-thaw cycles, fennel should be mulched heavily with straw or leaves to keep soil temperatures even and reduce the incidence of heaving.

If you are a tidy gardener who likes to remove old, dead growth for winter, you might be interested to learn that research indicates that allowing the dried stems of perennials to remain until the first spring growth emerges actually helps the plant survive winter's cold and increases its overall health. If you feel compelled to tidy up the fennel bed for winter, try to wait until the plant has died back completely before cutting the stems to the ground.

Fennel in the Kitchen

Fennel is an herb, spice, and vegetable all rolled into one beautiful plant. For thousands of years it has been a major component of Mediterranean, Middle Eastern, Indian, French, Chinese, and Italian cuisine. Although it has recently gained ground in fine dining establishments in the West, fennel is still underutilized by the average American cook.

Part of the problem with fennel is its relative lack of notoriety and availability in U.S. produce markets. Generally, one must live in a large metropolitan area to find fennel bulbs in the produce section with any regularity, and prepackaged fennel seed always takes low priority on grocery store spice racks. Without being exposed to it in real life, most people simply don't know what to do with fennel.

For starters, all parts of the fennel plant have a sweet, anise-like flavor, but the seeds are by far and away the most flavorful part. In fact, the seeds of fennel are used commercially as "licorice" flavoring in all kinds of products, from candy to liqueur to toothpaste. If you love red sauce, spaghetti, pizza, or other Italian foods, then you already like fennel seed.

Once I grew my own fennel seed, I found myself using it with abandon in dishes and drinks that I never would have imagined. Fennel seed is a nice addition to brewed black and green teas, fruit salads, desserts, and pastries. Try it on garlic or cheese breads just before toasting, or top your favorite yeast loaf with a healthy handful of fennel seeds for a real culinary treat. I also like to use fennel seed to sweeten bitter herbal teas or to flavor homemade liqueurs.

The least-used part of fennel is its fine, ferny leaves, which have a light anise flavor with a hint of green freshness thrown in for good measure. Because they are so pretty, fennel leaves are often used to garnish plated dishes and entrees, but the creative cook can dice or shred them before sprinkling them onto cold salads of fruit, vegetables, fish, and poultry. Fennel leaves also add a nice touch to plates of hot rice or pasta. Keep in mind that fennel leaves are always used fresh, because they don't retain their flavor when dried.

If you grow your own bulb fennel, the tender young stalks and the main bulb can be used in any way that you might use celery and in many ways that you would never use celery! The flesh is sweet and delicately crunchy, and has a fresh flavor that can't be found in any other vegetable. I particularly like chopped fennel in potato salad, tuna salad, coleslaw, and stir-fry. The bulb can be sectioned and filled with cheese, cream cheese, apples, dates, shrimp salad, or even peanut butter. The sky's the limit when it comes to dressing up these scrumptious stalks.

In addition to being good appetizers, the bulbs can be chopped, diced, shredded, or puréed and then added to soup, stew, broth, or consommé. They can be also be baked, broiled, braised, roasted, grilled, or caramelized and served or cooked with any type of meat or seafood that one might imagine.

With that kind of versatility, it's hard to imagine why fennel isn't a mainstay in every kitchen in America.

The Medicinal Side of Fennel

The ancient Romans believed that fennel seed reduced the appetite and controlled obesity. Today, it is well known for being a mild and reliable medicinal that has long been approved by the well-regarded German Commission E. It is a strong anti-inflammatory and antispasmodic, widely used for cramps, spasms, and menstrual pain. The mild estrogen-like action is used to regulate menstruation, increase the production of breast milk, and aid in menopausal symptoms.

Fennel tea is most often used to treat symptoms of cold and flu, such as cough, congestion, sore throat, fever, and muscle pain. It is known to strengthen and tone the digestive system, making it a beneficial herb in treating dyspepsia, indigestion, flatulence, heartburn, colic, and lower abdominal pain.

The seeds of fennel can be chewed as a mild numbing agent for temporary relief of minor pain caused by mouth sores or burning mouth syndrome. The slightly mucilaginous texture can also bring relief from dry mouth, ease a sore throat, and freshen the breath.

In general, fennel is a gentle and effective medicinal, but as with all things, there are some people who should not use this herb in medicinal doses without consulting their health care professional first. People who are suffering from chronic liver disease, hepatitis, epilepsy, or estrogen-dependent cancer and those taking ciprofloxacin should avoid using fennel altogether.

As a customary precaution, women who are pregnant or lactating should consult their herbalist or health care professional before using fennel medicinally. In addition, anyone known to have allergic reactions to carrots, celery, or other plants in the parsley family should avoid contact with fennel.

The pure essential oil of fennel is primarily used for external applications only after being diluted and should *never* be used internally without the supervision of a professional. If you use the essential oil of fennel, always keep it locked away from small hands. Less than one teaspoon (five ml) of this very concentrated oil can cause severe contact dermatitis, vomiting, seizure, hallucinations, pulmonary edema, and possibly death.

Heating an herbal decoction or infusion of fennel seed and breathing in the steam brings quick relief to those suffering from sinus or chest congestion by moisturizing a dry throat and nasal passages and by acting as a decongestant. Drinking a cup of fennel tea also helps reduce dry mucus in the mouth, which is especially helpful during bouts of flu.

Fennel is a natural conditioner, and when paired with apple cider vinegar, it can't be beat for softening the hair and adding body and shine. To prepare a hair rinse, simply run a cooled infusion or decoction of fennel seed through the hair into a shallow basin. Repeat the process several times before allowing the rinse to dry in the hair. Apply this treatment two to three times a week for best effect.

Glycerin- or vinegar-based tinctures are especially nice in products for dry, itchy skin or scalp, and adding a glycerin tincture of fennel to any homemade or store-bought product will make it more moisturizing.

In the end, fennel is a wonderful and gentle medicinal, an extraordinarily versatile vegetable and spice, and a tall, graceful herb that should be planted and used much more often than it is. Of course, if you love butterflies, plant a few extra fennel plants for the black swallowtail butterfly larvae to feed on and you'll have plenty of beautiful flying flowers to brighten all of your summer days.

Jill Henderson *is an artist, author, and world traveler with a penchant for wild edible and medicinal plants, culinary herbs, and nature ecology. She has written three books, including* The Healing Power of Kitchen Herbs: Growing and Using Nature's Remedies, A Journey of Seasons: A Year in the Ozarks High Country, *and* The Garden Seed Saving Guide: Seed Saving for Everyone.

A lifelong organic gardener and seed saver with a passion for sustainable agriculture and local food production, Jill presents workshops to teach gardeners about the detrimental impacts of bio-engineered food crops and how to grow and save open-pollinated and heirloom seeds.

Jill also writes and edits Show Me Oz *(ShowMeOz.wordpress.com), a weekly blog filled with gardening and seed-saving tips, homesteading wisdom, edible and medicinal plants, nature, and more. She is a regular contributor to* Llewellyn's Herbal Almanac, Acres USA, *and the* Permaculture Activist.

In her spare time, Jill is a professional artist specializing in custom pet portraits and wildlife art. You can view some of her work at ForeverPetPortraits.wordpress.com. Jill and her husband, Dean, live and work in the heart of the rugged Ozark Mountains.

Highland Heather &
Wild Thyme

❧ By Esthamarelda McNevin ❧

The highland cultures of Scotland revere the symbiotic relationship between wild heather and thyme, especially when it comes to the country herb garden. The pair is featured strongly as an emblem of romantic pastoral autonomy, in part because they wander, spread, and otherwise trail through unintended spaces. These companions are traditionally planted along stone walls and pathways. They also act as a dramatic and colorful ground cover used in cottage landscaping. With a wide range of varieties available, these two iconic flowering herbs make for an amorous consortium in the garden.

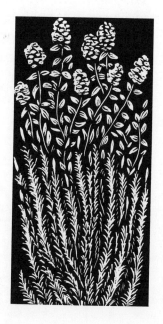

Along with the thistle, heather and thyme can be found on everything from kitschy tourist tea towels to music boxes that chime out Francis McPeake's famous 1957 folk tune. The catchy ballad, "Wild Mountain Thyme," was based almost entirely on Robert Tannahill's 1821 poem "The Braes of Balquhither." This dreamy and romantic Scottish ode to the glad innocence of rustic escapism and highland courtship is evocative of the summer season and countryside values.

In and among the ceaseless invasions and bloody clan wars that speckle Scotland's highland history with its brutal heroes, a wild and honest love of the craggy landscape prevailed through a deep appreciation of ecology, gardening, and cottage agriculture. It's not hard to see why, either. Travel magazines and blogs are filled with decadent photography showcasing the heather-filled hills of the Scottish moorlands. In this ancient glacial landscape, the purple majesty of flowering *Calluna vulgaris* (Ericaceae) has been forever bound both medicinally and ideologically to rambling thyme.

The ecology of Scotland has molded itself around long, cold winters and the torrential weather systems of the North Sea. Both heather and thyme thrive best in such dramatic and fast-changing conditions, especially when they are bedded down or clutched under cover for the winter. During the spring and summer months, they are also predisposed to full sun, making them exceptionally fast spreading when used in landscaping as meadow cover. Both heather and thyme thrive in well-drained acidic soil and absorb moisture and nutrients best when they are received from daily tidal and lakeland fog systems. As a result, they create mutually beneficial and resilient root structures when planted as companions.

The benefits of flowering herbs in the garden far outweigh their sometimes-finicky nature. Until they are established, both heather and thyme are prone to disease and rot if they are over or underwatered. They prefer to be watered twice daily at the exact same times. A break in this routine while heather shrubs are young will cause immature suckers to die back, or limit flower production and the development of new growth.

Nearly all culinary herbs must be harvested regularly or their first run of flowers will go to seed. The loss of nutrients from the leaves results in fat, juicy seeds destined for life, as well as a diminished flavor resulting in poor herb quality. Pruning often will prevent this. Likewise, heather flowers should be snipped back to control growth and the direction of their spread. Both herbs thrive in prepared sandy beds as well as patio containers.

Although cultivating perennial companion plants in the garden can take some time and careful attention, it does have its long-term rewards when it comes to soil building and cottage landscaping. Not to mention, every good chef knows that fresh herbs make all the difference in the kitchen.

Having heather flowers for tea and thyme for savory dishes on hand for the season can really be a financial blessing. Being able to store your own herbs for winter is a wonderful way to live more sustainably and to share the wealth of your garden throughout the year with the ones you love. The basic cultivation information for both heather and thyme is provided next, along with a few harvesting tips and recipe ideas. Try your hand at nurturing these age-old flowering herbs, and let the wild passion of the highlands fill your garden with the world enough, and time for romance.

Heather

Heather belongs to the Ericaceae family, which also includes cranberry, blueberry, huckleberry, azalea, and rhododendron. It is a flowering evergreen shrub that is native to the Mediterranean, Northern Europe, and Scotland. Heather grows to a height of eighteen to thirty-four inches by four feet wide. It is a hardy perennial with wood stems, small bell-shaped flowers, and tiny needle leaves. It grows in zones 5–7 and thrives in acidic, sandy peat moss soil. Heather requires consistent scheduled watering once or twice daily. Lightly soak and then mist each plant daily.

Heather provides a dramatic and colorful palate when used as a wide border or landscape filler. Starts are best purchased from a garden supply center or are cleaved from the root ball of existing shrubs. The matted mithril root system gives it a strong hold on the cold, sandy peat soil of northern climates and the rock face cliffs of the Mediterranean, marking heather as a renowned splash of color, often found in seemingly desolate lands.

In the lawn, this shrub serves as fast-growing field cover, which requires little to no care if placed near a body of water or a naturally occurring seasonal drainage corridor. This plant is most beloved once it is established in staggering rows or masses. The fluid contours of sprawling flowers take on a mystical and dreamy quality when moved by the wind. This effect lends an ambiance of highland romance to any garden.

Highlands and Moorlands

The Ericaceae family is divided into two primary groups: *Erica*, the delicate yet colorful Mediterranean moorland heaths, and

Calluna vulgaris, the hardy highland heathers. Both are flowering evergreen shrubs that add color and fragrance to any allotment. As low-maintenance plants, they thrive best (once established) when left to take over an area prone to morning dew and condensation. Both species require the same relative care and acidic soil condition; creating a soil pH of 6–7.5 is essential. Loved by many gardeners because they act as soil-building contributors when they are grown in mounded groups of five or more, both heather and heath are drought-intolerant and require scheduled watering until they are established. Heathers do best when they are misted or able to draw ambient dew twice daily.

Of the two, *Erica*, or heath, is native to Africa and the Mediterranean. It will die back seasonally in extreme humid or frigid conditions, and when planting, this species prefers crushed seashells to peat moss. The small needle-like leaves conceal bell-shaped flowers that range in hue from blush pink to deep purple. This shrub is tolerant of nearly all soils and will spread best in depleted and neglected areas of the sunny yard or garden.

Erica varieties have a greater tendency to grow into small trees when they are not delicately pruned just after flowering. Heath is planted in fall one month before the first frost and is rarely fertilized. This is because most soil conditioners will encourage open gangly stalk growth, causing the root mound to focus nutrient absorption on primary shoots.

Calluna vulgaris is the original heather of the northern lands of Scotland and Europe. It is favored as far north as zone 3, where cultivators clutch and insulate the plant throughout the dormant winters with pine mulch and straw. Its blooms feature leaf-guarded corolla, where whorls of petals are encased by the green leaves from below. This gives *Calluna* varieties a two-tone color quality and more densely packed buds. For this reason, they are greatly favored for use in teas and are a common seasonal garnish in Scottish cakes and pastries.

Harvesting Heather

From midsummer to early fall, begin lightly pruning back blossoms. Take care never to overprune, as this will cause dieback in other areas of the shrub. Stop pruning a full month prior to the first frost of autumn to allow the shrub time to prepare for dormancy. To preserve the flowers, bundle and hang heather sprigs in a warm, dry location. Remove as needed for use in dried flower boxes and craft projects. Heather springs make a lovely addition to dried bouquets, oil bottles, and hand-milled soaps. The dried flowers are commonly used in potpourri blends and can be strung throughout the home as festive summer and autumn decorations.

For use in the kitchen, harvest heather and heath just after flowering has begun, when all the buds are not yet open. Separate the flowers and leaves from the stem, and dry them on different wire mesh racks. The flowers make a lovely tea that has been used to promote kidney and bladder health for centuries by Scottish herbalists. The leaves can be used in baked goods and vegetable dishes, where they lend a sweet, slightly bitter and evergreen flavor, similar in profile to fresh rosemary and juniper. This is often added to northern river fish and grassland grouse dishes, which are pan-seared, broiled, glazed, or garnished with heather honey.

Thyme

Thyme belongs to the Lamiaceae family and is related to mint. It is a flowering evergreen shrub. *Thymus vulgaris* is native to Africa and Mediterranean. It grows to a height of six to fifteen inches. Thyme is a hardy perennial with woody stems, small tube flowers, and silver/gray-green leaves. It grows in zones 5–9 and thrives in alkaline, sandy soil with crushed seashells. Thyme requires consistent scheduled watering once or twice daily. Lightly soak and then mist each plant daily.

Thyme makes for an excellent addition to any sunny border and spreads quickly when planted as low-level bed filling or ground cover. Scottish cottage gardeners favor thyme between path stones and steps, as well as in window boxes and patio containers, because it companions well with other flowering culinary herbs, peppers, and most ornamental grasses. The petite two-lipped tubular blossoms range in color from subtle pink to deep purple. They flower from early to late summer, attracting bumblebees to help pollinate the garden.

Seed, Soil, and Water

Thyme requires full sunlight. This age-old favorite does best in soils that offer unrestricted drainage and an alkaline environment with a pH of 7.0. Adding a bit of garden lime to the prepared bed or large potting container, along with a teaspoon of fish emulsion each spring, will help to bring on more blossoms. Top mulching with sand, lime stone gravel, and peat moss will additionally encourage the drainage that thyme needs to thrive. When overwatered, all flowering culinary herbs are very susceptible to root rot and insect infestation. Choosing a location with good air circulation is essential.

Seeds are best sown inside and require a hygienic humid environment with an ambient temperature regulated at 70°F (21°C) for germination. Once sprouts are six inches, they can be moved to a prepared spring bed or container once all chance of frost has passed. Plant them one foot apart and keep the area weeded to prevent competition for nutrients. Prepare the bed or container carefully to be sure that the soil is composed of 50 percent rich top soil, 30 percent sand, and 20 percent crushed sea shells and will mimic the nutrient-rich soil system of the Mediterranean. Mulch the topsoil around the shoots when they begin to show additional growth, about a week or so after transplanting them outdoors.

Harvesting Thyme

In zones 5–9, take care to stop clipping all evergreen shrubs like thyme at least one month before the first frost, as this will allow the plant the chance to prepare for autumn's colder weather. Control the growth and spread of your little patch of thyme by pinching back a few early spring buds to encourage bushing growth later on during the peak of the season. Though this species requires tender care in the first two years of cultivation, once it is established thyme will take over if it is not regularly and lovingly pruned.

Collecting a little bit of thyme habitually with clippers will help keep plants growing well throughout the season. Always harvest from the points of new growth, and never clip the lower portions of the leafless woody stem or you may introduce bacteria into the root mound from the stalk. Trimming thyme from its nether regions like this will encourage dieback. Once your thyme has matured into its location, when it is two or three years old, liberally prune after the last frost of early spring has passed.

Having thyme on hand can prove inspiring when it comes to cooking up pasta and fish dishes. Store your clippings for up to two weeks by keeping them in a glass herb vase or sake flask on a shelf in the refrigerator. Change the water every couple of days to keep them fresh. If you can't use them fast enough, bind a few sprigs together and hang them to dry or strip the leaves from the stem and place them on a wire mesh or in a closed paper lunch sack. Hang this in a pantry until the leaves are fully dehydrated, then store your homegrown thyme in a kitchen herb jar or give samples away as a culinary gift.

Recipe

Heather & Thyme Tea

Victorian teahouses loved to specialize in local flavors like heather tea. Many recipes can be found, and most highland teas are sweetened with heather honey as a general rule of thumb. This tea is light and subtly floral, with herbal overtones and a robust aroma. It is best served with raspberry scones and crème custard.

Assemble:

1 teaspoon dry heather flowers

1 pinch fresh thyme

2 rose hips, crushed

1 teaspoon heather honey

Combine all of the listed ingredients in a tea infuser ball and steep for 5 minutes in 4 cups (24 fl. oz.) of boiled water. Strain and serve hot. Enjoy!

Garden Project

Barrel of Balquhither: Large Container Planting of Heather & Thyme

Francis McPeake wrote his famous 1957 folk tune "Wild Mountain Thyme," oddly enough, while living in Ireland. It became a beloved ballad in part because it romanticizes freedom as an inherently bucolic bliss, which often has more to do with love than we care to admit. Likewise, Robert Tannahill's 1821 poem "The Braes of Balquhither" pays tribute to the wild ecosystem of the heather-hilled highlands, depicted in song as the secluded utopia of the freedom fighter. As a Scottish descendant, it fills me with both highland pride and gardening pleasure to companion heather and thyme throughout the garden in the name of highland love and human liberty.

These herbs companion famously well together when regularly pruned and planted out on a sunny back deck or patio. Container gardening can be a fun and dramatic way to display flowering herbs like heather and thyme. The benefit of cultivating culinary herbs near to the kitchen is that they can be gathered throughout the season quickly, by just popping out the back door with a trusty pair of secateurs. Back porch and outdoor spaces also come alive when herbs fill the space with flowers and perfume the air with all the ambiance of the blooming bounty of free, highland love.

Once they have known the glory of the season, large planters and containers should be stored for the winter in a garden shed or insulated with straw-stuffed burlap casings, sometime during those last days of summer. This is to help container perennials withstand the autumn evening drop in temperature. Gardeners must insulate delicate root structures kept above ground throughout the impending season of dormancy, because container plants haven't the natural insulation created by ground cover and soil mass.

Assemble:

A 20-inch large cedar planting barrel

8 large sedimentary rocks

Sand

Fine river gravel

Crushed seashells

Rich top soil to fill

1 heather plant

4 thyme plants

Peat moss

Limestone gravel

Line the bottom of the barrel with large rocks to provide increased drainage. Cover with one inch of sand. Then fill the container with two inches of gravel and crushed seashells. On top of this add another inch of sand. In a separate container, mix equal parts of rich top soil and sand and then fill the container with this mixture. Plant a single heather shrub in the center, and circle the thyme around the edge. When you are done planting, mix equal parts of sand and peat moss, and then apply this to the top layer of the container. Finally, sprinkle the surface with a handful of limestone gravel.

Heather and thyme both love consistent morning and evening water cycles, but like all large garden containers, lightly soaking and then misting each plant daily will conserve both water and nutrients. Container plants will leach nutrients when they are overwatered, and both heather and thyme are suscep-tible to root putrefaction, especially when left to standing water and poor air circulation. Take care to apply a fertilizer of one tablespoon fish emulsion diluted in one gallon of water every six weeks as needed for sustained growth. Treat transplanted shrubs and herbs with tender care until the container is estab-lished. Then harvest and enjoy!

For More Information

American Heather Society, www.northamericanheathersociety
.org.

Darwin, Tess. *The Scots Herbal: The Plant Lore of Scotland.*
Edinburgh: Mercat Press, 1997.

Milliken, William, and Sam Bridgewater. *Flora Celtica: Plants and People in Scotland.* Edinburgh: Birlinn, 2004.

Bateman, Helen. *The Practical Gardener's Encyclopedia.*
San Francisco, CA: Fog City, 2000.

Esthamarelda McNevin *(Missoula, MT) is the founding Priestess and oracle of the Eastern Hellenistic magickal temple* Opus Aima Obscuræ *(OAO). In the greater community she works as a lecturer, baker, writer, organic gardener, and psychic intuitive and is co-owner of the metaphysical business Twigs & Brews. She also conducts pri-vate spiritual consultations, spirit intermediations, and Tarot read-ings for the greater Pagan community. Visit her at www.facebook .com/opusaimaobscurae.*

A Little Bit of Earth: An Overview of Amateur Gardening Options

⇲ By Emyme ⇱

Novice. Intermediate. Expert/ Master. You have decided to take up the tools and walk the garden path, or deviate from the path(s) previously chosen. Whatever the level of your experience, here are just a few of the reasons gardens may have taken center stage in your life.

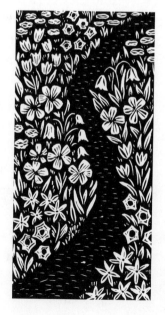

- You finally own your first home. After years of apartment living—limited to window boxes and potted plants on windowsills—you can create the garden of your dreams. The curb appeal is shabby, but it did not deter you from the purchase. In fact, this is an opportunity to make your mark, and landscaping advice is sorely needed.

- You have downsized to a smaller home for your empty nest, and have left behind the gardens you worked so hard to nurture. The need to start your gardens all over again is tempered by the reality of having a smaller space. Perhaps now is the time to concentrate on herbs.

- Your children or grandchildren are finally old enough, or still young enough, to discover the love of soil in their hands. Time, patience, and good weather conditions are needed, as well as smaller hoes and rakes and spades.

- You have retired from the nine-to-five workday and will now devote time to becoming more than just a casual weekend gardener. Roses, or orchids, or cacti grow especially well in your zone, and you have chosen to master them. Maybe now is the time to try for organic heirloom vegetables.

- Your move to a different climate / zone means everything you ever knew about plants in zone 1 has little or nothing to do with zone 10. You must start fresh, with no clue as to what will thrive in the garden of the home you now occupy.

- You notice that the new building down the road has been completed. A notice in the paper and a sign outside of the construction ask for volunteers to finish the landscaping. This feels like the nudge you need to expand from your own yard to the community.

- You wish to create a gardening co-op in your neighborhood. Every backyard is large enough to grow something, be it a few staked tomato plants or a row of zucchini. Whatever is grown will be shared with the three or five or eight families who agree to contribute.

For any of these or a dozen other reasons, you have decided, on a scale grand or miniature, to branch out. What is the first step in any of these endeavors, these scenarios? It is, of course, a trip to the local nursery, garden center, or even the big-box home store. The choices are many, confusing—where to start?

On a local level, there is almost always a garden club around every corner. In the heart of even the largest urban areas, there are nurseries. They will be in tune with local organizations and may sponsor clubs themselves. Even the big-box home improvement stores now have garden clubs, Home Depot in particular. Your neighborhood, county, and/or community libraries will definitely have information on whom to contact. Then there is the Internet: simply type "garden clubs" or "flower show" into your search engine of choice. The choices may be narrowed down from there. Often, websites for the national or international organization will have links to country, state, and local clubs. It's also possible to work in the other direction, with local clubs providing links to the umbrella organization that monitors/sponsors the smaller chapters.

It may seem as though you are being bombarded with choices, and from here you do indeed have more decisions to make. What type of gardening club are you looking for?

Some clubs meet in the evening, catering to those who work full time during the day. Others meet during the day on weekdays, perhaps catering to retired folks or taking advantage of the daylight hours to actually garden during the meetings. A gathering of like-minded souls with the title of "garden club" may also be simply a social group. Consider the extent of your competitive nature. Some clubs are formed for contests only:

who can grow the biggest or sweetest or prettiest or best-smelling/tasting plant, flower, or vegetable. Another consideration is that some clubs deal strictly with gardens from which food is grown, others with just flowers, and some combine the two. Depending on your inclination, you may have to do a little legwork to find a good fit. If the feel of the club is not right for you, do not stay. It will only discourage you. Members of a good club will be welcoming and inviting and open to all, no matter the level of experience.

An alternative entry into the community of amateur gardening is the local education system. For years, continuing education classes have been offered at local middle and high schools in the domestic arts and gardening, along with auto repair and metal and woodworking. Continuing education is a large and thriving enterprise. Look for classes that spotlight family involvement, which is an easy way to get the children involved or to volunteer your expertise. Community colleges and larger institutions of learning also offer courses, and not just in suburban and rural areas. Due to the growing popularity of city gardens and the importance of city dwellers having access to fresh healthy fruits and vegetables, many colleges help with the city gardens. There are courses that teach the history and the future of food. Some colleges offer degrees and hands-on classes that take students back to how gardening was two centuries ago, or imagine how it may be one hundred years from now.

Now, a few years down the road, you have decided to specialize in one thing: roses, violets, tulips, cactus, astilbe, or chrysanthemums. Pumpkins, apples, or holly. Topiaries or terrariums, dish gardens or rock gardens. The soil in your yard, the sun or shade on your gardens, the compost you nurture—everything has come together in a perfect combination to help you grow a perfect something. Now what do you do?

You would love to show this off. Your club associates, your classmates, your teachers, your students even—everyone tells you to join a competition. But how is that done? It appears to finally be the time to look into competitive flower shows. And why not start with one of the best? My personal experience has been with the Philadelphia Flower Show, sponsored by the Pennsylvania Horticultural Society. More than 185 years old and billed as "the largest indoor flower show in the world," it attracts tens of thousands of participants and visitors from all over the world.

The weather can be changeable and unpredictable in early March in center city Philadelphia. Parking is expensive, and you may have to walk a few blocks to get to the show. The trains are crowded but might get you closer. Hotels offer special packages. The city is busier than usual near the Pennsylvania Convention Center this time of year.

From the beginning of your journey, you will experience an endless number of lines of people: lines to get in the main doors, lines to buy your ticket or show your ticket, lines to get on the escalator or the elevator or to use the steps, lines to get into the showroom. When the doors suddenly open and you are engulfed in sight and sound and smell, it is a wonderful explosion to the senses.

Here is where your involvement with local garden clubs, or continuing education classes, or that college course on heirloom tomatoes will prove their worth. Much like any flower show on any scale, the Philadelphia Flower Show has an amateur section; gardeners bring in their best of the best, just one plant or flower for judging. This show provides amateurs a place to shine, right alongside the professionals.

Displays in recent years have included elaborate scenes—interpretated by professionals—utilizing fresh and living flowers and plants, from the smallest herb to the tallest tree; a series of front porches decorated by high school students; plus a series of mailboxes and window boxes done up by garden club members. Huge window dressings and miniature dioramas fascinate in turn.

Another section showcases framed artwork created with only dried flowers and leaves. Here, college students have re-created a garden from the eighteenth century exactly as it was, with fencing, greenhouse, and irrigation all supporting seeds dating back to the 1770s.

Finally, there are the vendors. Anything you may wish to purchase for your garden, be it equipment or decoration, can be found in the shopping section. There are plants and plant products, and also house and personal decoration, including jewelry, scarves, and home décor.

The last thing we need to consider on our journey is horticulture. Every gardener at every level, from the rank amateur to the seasoned professional, is a horticulturist. Horticulture is the cultivation of plants for use by humans, be it for reasons of basic survival (food and drink for nourishment, wood for homes and furniture) or simply for beauty. The diversity of the science and business of horticulture is staggering. Horticulture encompasses conservation and landscape restoration and design. Even the health care industry depends on horticulture.

Many, if not all, medicines start out as plant extracts. Physical and occupational gardening therapy provide soothing treatment. Few things calm us down faster than time spent puttering in the garden and working in the dirt. Horticulture contributes to society in such vast and diverse ways that it staggers the imagination.

If you are reading this almanac, you wish for or already have an all-encompassing connection to the natural world. Humans have a relationship with plants. It is up to the individual to choose the level of participation. You may choose to purchase all-natural supplies, while others choose to work only with the supplies they have personally grown. Some people work with plants from their own garden, bought and nurtured from four-inch pots, and some work only with their own plants grown directly from seed. There is a faction who limit themselves to what they find on nature walks, choosing to work with what is found or presented to them by nature.

One good thing about the decision to become more involved with nature and the earth is this: whether you shop at the local supermarket plant section, the farmers' market down the road, the larger nursery two towns over, or the big-box store by the mall, you never have to apologize for or explain your choices. Plant lovers are welcomed everywhere. You will also find much encouragement and answers to all your questions. Wherever in the world you live, whatever your level of participation with horticulture, with nature— seek out the flower shows, the courses and classes, the garden clubs. You will not be disappointed. Most likely, you will be inspired to travel further along that garden path.

For More Information

Pennsylvania Horticultural Society. *The Philadelphia Flower Show*. Charleston, SC: Arcadia Publishing, 2014.

References

Philadelphia Flower Show, theflowershow.org.

Royal Horticultural Society, www.rhs.org.uk.

Harrogate Flower Show, www.flowershow.org.uk.

Melbourne International Flower and Garden Show, http://melbflowershow.com.au.

National Garden Clubs, gardenclub.org.

The Herb Society of America, herbsociety.org.

Emyme, *an eclectic solitary, resides in a multi-generation, multi-cat household in Southern New Jersey—concentrating on candle spells, garden spells, and kitchen witchery. In addition to writing poetry and prose about strong women of mythology and fairy tales, Emyme is creating a series of articles on bed & breakfasts from the point of view of the over-fifty-five, single, female, Wiccan traveler. Please send questions or comments to catsmeow24@verizon.net.*

The Many Faces of Monarda

✍ By Jill Henderson ✍

There is nothing quite as enchanting as a chance encounter with a thriving patch of beautiful, medicinal *Monarda* in bloom. The near-electric colors of these common garden plants are sure to light up any spot in the landscape and dazzle the unsuspecting eye with multitudes of large, shaggy, upright flowers. And should you encounter *Monarda* in the wild, there's a good chance that you will have been led to it by the sound of buzzing bees.

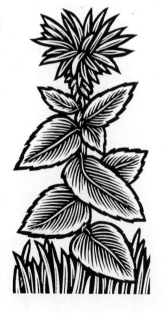

The Name Says It All

The most common species of *Monarda* are often collectively referred to as beebalm, but depending on where you live, they might be called any number of common names, including oswego tea, horsemint, and wild bergamot—all of which are the common names for various species belonging to the genus *Monarda*.

North America boasts a whopping seventeen native species of *Monarda* and multitudes of named cultivars. In this article, I will refer to the plants in this genus simply as *Monarda*, unless I am referring to a specific species. The name *Monarda* was given to this genus in honor of Nicolás Monardes, a Spanish botanist and physician who wrote about New World plants.

Monarda belong to the Lamiaceae (mint) family of plants. They are herbaceous perennials and annuals that have three- to six-inch lance-shaped leaves growing in opposite pairs along a square, slightly hairy stem—a classic mint family trait. The leaves also tend to be slightly hairy and have lightly toothed margins. A few species have lemon- or mint-scented leaves, but most smell very much like oregano, another mint family member.

Like other mint family plants, *Monarda* have long, tubular flowers that are divided into a narrow upper lip and a wider lower lip, perfectly designed to entice bee landings. Each blossom, or inflorescence, is made up of many individual flowers, which are grouped in one- to three-inch clusters at the ends of stems (terminate) or along the upper leaf axils, depending on the species.

Flowers range in color from soft pink to deep purple to fire-engine red. Some species have cream to yellow flowers with purple spots. There's even a cultivar with flowers the color of orange sherbet! And because each inflorescence contains a multitude of individual flowers that open slowly over an extended period of time, *Monarda* provide a long-lasting floral display in the garden.

The two species of *Monarda* that are most often encountered in the wild are wild bergamot (*Monarda fistulosa*), which has rich, purple-pink flowers, and beebalm (*Monarda didyma*), whose flowers are an electric shade of red. Both species make excellent garden specimens and, along with their wild counterparts, have long been used by breeders to create new and interesting cultivated varieties.

The chart on the next page lists the currently recognized species of *Monarda* in North America. It does not include named cultivars, which number in the hundreds. And because *Monarda* plants naturally and easily hybridize in the wild, new species can appear at any time.

You may have noticed that many *Monarda* share similar common names that include the words beebalm, horsemint, and bergamot. The name "beebalm" is a natural for *Monarda*, because they do indeed attract a plethora of bees. But the use of the name "horsemint" is a little more confusing. After an extensive search of botanical epithets, I found no basis for the name in either Latin or Greek.

However, almost all of the *Monarda* species referred to as horsemint appear to prefer dry, sandy locations and were most likely encountered in fields or pastures where horses continually grazed and thus were called horsemint for lack of a better name. Either that, or some people found that the leaves of certain *Monarda* species smelled like a sweaty horse. I prefer the first scenario.

The name "bergamot" may also seem as odd as "horsemint," since true bergamot is actually the inedible fruit of a citrus tree known as bergamot orange (*Citrus aurantium* ssp. *bergamia*). Grown since ancient times in regions of southern

Species of Monarda	Common Name	Flower Color	Habitat
PERENNIALS			
M. bartlettii	Bartlette's Beebalm, Bartlett's Monarda	Purple to magenta	WD, FS-PSh, Mildew Resist
M. bradburiana	Eastern Beebalm, Wild Bergamot, Horsemint, Bradbury Beebalm	Lilac to white with purple spots	WD sand rocky, FS- PSh, DT
M. clinopodia	White Bergamot	White to light pink	MWD, average soils, FS-PSh
M. didyma	Oswego Tea, Red Bergamot, Scarlet Beebalm	Red	MWD, rich loam, FS-PSh
M. fistulosa	Wild Bergamot, Beebalm	White, pink, or purple	MWD, FS-PSh, DT
M. lindheimeri	Lindheimer's Beebalm	White	MWD, FS-PSh, DT
M. menthaefolia	Mintleaf Bergamot, Oregano de la Sierra	Bright pink	MWD, FS-PSh
M. pringlei	Lemon Horsemint, Pringle's Beebalm, Pringle's Bergamot, Dwarf Beebalm	Red to bright pink	WD, Part Shade, Mildew Resist
M. russeliana	Redpurple Beebalm, Russell's Horsemint	Purple-pink	MWD, S-PSh

Species	Common Names	Flower Color	Growing Conditions
M. viridissima	Green Beebalm, Green Horsemint	White to pink with red spots, showy bracts	Dry sandy loam, FS-PSh, DT
M. fruticulosa	Spotted Beebalm, Shrubby Horsemint, South Texas Beebalm	White to light pink	Dry sandy loam, FS-PSh, DT
M. media	Purple Beebalm, Purple Bergamot	Reddish pink to purple	MWD, Rich loam, FS-PSh
ANNUALS			
M. citriodora	Lemon Beebalm, Purple Horsemint, Lemon Mint, Plains Horsemint, Lemon Horsemint	White to lilac, purple leaf bracts	WD rocky sand, FS-PSh, DT
M. clinopodioides	Basil Beebalm, East Texas Horsemint	Soft pink	WD sandy clay, FS-PSh, DT
M. pectinata	Pony Beebalm, Horsemint, Plains Beebalm, Spotted Beebalm, Pagoda Plant	Purple with white spots, purple bracts	WD sandy, FS-PSh, DT
M. punctata	Spotted Beebalm, Spotted Horsemint, Dotted Horsemint	Creamy yellow with purple spots, showy purple bracts	WD sandy, FS-PSh, DT

WD = well-drained, MWD = moist well-drained, DT = drought-tolerant, FS-PSh = full sun to part shade

Italy, southern France, and the Ivory Coast of Africa, the bergamot orange tree is grown exclusively for the volatile oils found in the skin of the fruit, which are used in perfumery and as a distinct flavoring for products like Earl Grey tea. But the use of the name "bergamot" to describe some *Monarda* species most likely came about when early European settlers, who no longer had access to true bergamot, found the plant's scent pleasingly similar.

More Than Just Beautiful

Of course, the leaves and flowers of all *Monarda* species are edible to one degree or another, though some are obviously more pleasant than others. Carefully dried, the leaves of *M. didyma* and *M. fistulosa* can be readily used with, or in place of, either oregano or marjoram. I find the herb to be a nice addition to mixed spice blends such as Italian seasoning, and as a substitute for black pepper. The leaves' strong yet subtle flavor goes well with any type of meat, poultry, or fish and is most excellent on roasted potatoes and root vegetables. The lemon-flavored *Monarda* species, such as *M. citriodora*, can be used like lemon thyme on fish, chicken, seafood, and pasta. The lemony monardas also make a lovely hot tea.

The flowers of *Monarda* are also edible and are most welcome in green salads and cold fruit salads. When added to finished bottles of herbed vinegar, the individual flowers of *Monarda* impart a subtle flavor and add a pretty visual touch.

In addition to being quite edible, naturally occurring species of *Monarda*—particularly *M. didyma* and *M. fistulosa*—are tried and true medicinals. Throughout this article, I have purposely reinforced the fact that *Monarda* are similar to other mint family members in order to stress their value as both culinary herbs and medicinal plants. Medicinally speaking, *Monarda* can be safely used in every way that plants in the *Origanum*, *Thymus*, and *Mentha* genera are used.

Herbalists widely recommend and use native *M. didyma* for medicinal purposes because it has been shown to have the highest concentrations of volatile oils. If you choose to use another native species or a cultivated hybrid, be aware that it may not be as active medicinally.

Because of their relationship to oregano and thyme, most *Monarda* species contain naturally high levels of thymol and carvacrol—two biocide compounds known to help reduce the incidence of bacterial resistance to antibiotics like penicillin. Thymol has also been shown to be effective against fungal infections, specifically those involved in cases of drug-resistant *Candida* infections.

Recent research indicates that thymol is also showing great promise as a strong antimutagenic and antitumor agent, which may help treat or prevent some types of cancer. And while thymol is soluble in water (as in a tea or decoction), the medicinal properties of the leaves are much more potent when tinctured.

Proven as an antimicrobial biocide compound, thymol is used commercially as an antiseptic in many commercial mouthwashes. To help ease and heal a sore throat, toothache, or mouth sore, simply rinse regularly with a strong decoction of the fresh or dried leaves of common *Monarda*.

To ease the symptoms of common ailments such as gas, nausea, and colds or flu accompanied by fever or sore throat, slowly sip one to two cups of freshly brewed *Monarda* tea each day. To make the tea more palatable, sweeten it with a bit of honey.

With its antiseptic and anesthetic properties, a strong decoction of *Monarda* applied with a cotton ball or moist compress is very useful in preventing infections of minor wounds, rashes, scrapes, and cuts. The same strong decoction can be used as a wash or soak to treat fungal infections of the hands and feet, and can double as a rinse to stimulate hair growth.

For medicinal and culinary uses, the leaves of *Monarda* can be collected anytime, but the medicinal value is highest just as the plant begins to bloom. Fresh leaves are often a little bitter-tasting, but drying helps to sweeten them. Harvest leaves by cutting the stems with a sharp pair of scissors just above a pair of leaves. Be sure to leave several inches of leafy stem above the crown so the plant can regenerate new leaves.

There are two ways to dry leaves for later use. The first is to remove all the leaves from their stems and spread them out on a screen to dry. The other is to tie the ends of several stems together into loose, airy bunches and hang them in a shady area until the leaves are crisp. Whole leaves can be safely stored in an airtight jar in a dark, cool place for up to six months. The flowers can be set aside and used fresh or dried.

To make *Monarda* tea, place one to two tablespoons of dried herb in one cup of just-boiled water. Cover and steep for ten to fifteen minutes. To prepare a strong, healing decoction for external applications, simply double the amount of leaves and allow the brew to steep off of the heat for one to several hours.

Fresh leaf tinctures are easy to make using a 1:2 ratio (one part leaf to two parts drinking alcohol). Allow to steep for several weeks before straining and bottling. The typical dose for *Monarda* tinctures is four to six milliliters added to six ounces of water and taken up to three times per day. Teas, decoctions, and tinctures can all be used directly on the skin or added to herbal preparations like salves, ointments, lotions, and shampoos.

Monarda in the Garden

Monarda is an absolute stunner in its natural habitat, which makes it an exemplary addition to naturalized areas and wild-flower gardens. Yet it shines equally bright in cultivated flower, vegetable, and herb gardens, where it attracts a plethora of pollinating bees, beautiful butterflies, and busy hummingbirds.

Some gardeners report that *M. fistulosa* is the easiest species to start from seed, but all *Monarda* species will readily self-sow when given the right environment. The only catch is that the seeds of almost every species require a period of cold moist stratification before they will germinate.

For those gardeners who purchase their seeds from commercial seed sources or nurseries, manual stratification is not necessary. Most seed houses stratify their seeds prior to distribution. However, seeds that have been collected from the wild or from cultivated gardens will need to be stratified, which is easily accomplished by sowing the seeds outdoors, anytime from late fall to early winter.

In the spring, thin young seedlings that have at least one pair of true leaves to stand six to eight inches apart, with a final spacing of eighteen to twenty-four inches, depending on the species. The same spacing guidelines apply to potted nursery stock and root divisions. Be sure to keep young and newly transplanted plants well watered until they are firmly established.

Keep in mind that not all *Monarda* like the same growing conditions. Some species thrive in full sun and rich soil, while others require partial shade and sandy soil. Refer to the previous chart for the preferred growing conditions of each

Monarda species. If unsure of the species, plant *Monarda* in an area that receives early morning sun and late afternoon shade and provide it with average, well-drained soil.

Like other mint family members, *Monarda* spread by seed and an extensive system of shallow, rhizomatous roots. Take care to give perennial *Monarda* plenty of room in the garden, and plan to divide the plants every few years to keep them in check. Dividing also helps prevent diseases of the root system and generates lots of new plants for friends and family.

If left to their own devices, some of the more common *Monarda* species can grow very tall and lanky, making them top-heavy while in bloom. To help keep large plants tidy and upright, trim an inch or two off the very tips of the plants in mid-spring when they are ten to twelve inches tall and again when spent flowers are removed. This also helps the plant to produce more flowers.

Like other mints, *Monarda* are prone to powdery mildew during hot, dry spells. To help prevent this disease, avoid over-crowding and overhead watering, keep soils constantly and evenly moist, and remove infected foliage immediately. In the fall, cut plants almost to the ground and remove the debris from the garden. This not only helps prevent future bouts of mildew but helps prevent the spread of rust, which occasion-ally plagues *Monarda*.

Long used as a companion planting in organic gardens, *Monarda* does in fact have natural insecticidal qualities due to its high levels of thymol, which has been identified as a class of hydrocarbon monoterpene that is also found in common thyme. Not only do these terpenes attract good bugs, such as bees and butterflies, but they also have the ability to repel or kill bad bugs, such as the larvae of the Colorado potato beetle when a leaf decoction is sprayed on plants.

As an organic pesticide, thymol is very short lived in soil (five days) and water (sixteen days), which helps prevent intrusion into waterways. And according to the U.S. Environmental Protection Agency Office of Pesticide Programs, "No unreasonable adverse effects on humans or the environment are anticipated from aggregate exposure to thymol."[1]

As if that weren't enough, deer and other browsers dislike the smell and taste of *Monarda*, and will leave these beautiful natives untouched.

No matter what you prefer to call them, *Monarda* plants are blessed with an incredible array of attributes that will more than pay for themselves in beauty and functionality. If you haven't tried *Monarda* in your garden before, now is a perfect time to start.

Endnote

1. U.S. Environmental Protection Agency Office of Pesticide Programs, "THYMOL 5-methyl-2-isopropyl-1-phenol (PC Code 080402)," www.epa.gov/pesticides/chem_search/reg_actions/registration/decision_PC-080402_23-Mar-06.pdf.

Jill Henderson *is an artist, author, and world traveler with a penchant for wild edible and medicinal plants, culinary herbs, and nature ecology. She has written three books, including* The Healing Power of Kitchen Herbs: Growing and Using Nature's Remedies, A Journey of Seasons: A Year in the Ozarks High Country, *and* The Garden Seed Saving Guide: Seed Saving for Everyone.

A lifelong organic gardener and seed saver with a passion for sustainable agriculture and local food production, Jill presents workshops to teach gardeners about the detrimental impacts of bio-engineered food crops and how to grow and save open-pollinated and heirloom seeds.

Jill also writes and edits Show Me Oz (ShowMeOz.wordpress .com), a weekly blog filled with gardening and seed-saving tips, homesteading wisdom, edible and medicinal plants, nature, and more. She is a regular contributor to Llewellyn's Herbal Almanac, Acres USA, and the Permaculture Activist.

In her spare time, Jill is a professional artist specializing in custom pet portraits and wildlife art. You can view some of her work at ForeverPetPortraits.wordpress.com. Jill and her husband, Dean, live and work in the heart of the rugged Ozark Mountains.

Permaculture for Herbalists

☙ By Elizabeth Barrette ❧

Permaculture is a set of principles and practices that use nature as inspiration for agriculture and landscaping. Instead of a short-term, separate approach to growing plants, this method takes a long-term, integrated perspective. The result is a cohesive system that supports many of its own needs while producing abundant materials for human enjoyment.

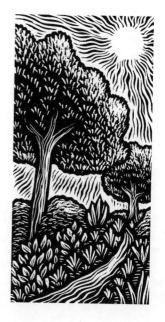

The idea behind permaculture is to create a permanent community of life forms, so it uses very little tilling and sowing. Once the plants are established, they are left in place, protected by mulch. Dense, layered plantings reduce the opportunity for weeds. Nutrient gatherers minimize fertilizer. Natural repellants in leaves and roots discourage pests, which are also controlled by beneficial wildlife.

When designing a permaculture landscape, work from the large scale to the small scale. Use patterns such as water flow to tell you where things belong: sun-loving herbs in a hot, dry space, and water-tolerant ones where it gets soggy after a rain. Integrate the parts of the system so they work together. One tree provides shade, wood, nuts or fruit, and wildlife habitat. Dandelions underneath bring up deep minerals, provide salad greens, and attract pollinators. Together they are healthier than either would be alone.

Make little changes that will grow slowly over time rather than trying to do too much at once. A single herb bed makes an ideal introduction to permaculture as a concept. Conversely, it helps to diversify your plantings. If something goes wrong in one, the others may still be thriving. Use the edges of the landscape to your advantage; nature is most diverse and active in marginal areas. Wildlife therefore gravitates to borders.

A permaculture gardener observes and interacts with the landscape. For magical folks, this provides an opportunity to attune yourself with nature, the spirits, and the elements. They will show you what to do if you pay attention. Like nature, a good permaculture system will catch and store energy, wasting nothing. For example, rainwater may be captured in a rain garden or swales instead of making a nuisance of itself as runoff. Use renewable resources; minimize the input and outflow to keep everything cycling within the system. When problems arise, gently adjust the permaculture to take care of itself; you may need to encourage more insect predators to control pests or add mulch plants to deter weeds.

The garden also produces many yields. For an herb garden-er, this may include medicinal and culinary items, craft supplies such as dyes or dried flowers, wildlife to enjoy, and spare time no longer gobbled up by garden chores.

Companion Planting

Companion planting is a basic concept of permaculture that often appears on a small scale in other gardening plans. The goal is to combine plants that support each other's needs while separating those that have a negative impact on each other. This reduces the amount of human care required to keep the garden healthy.

Consider the shape of plants in companion planting. Choose ones whose root systems will not compete. Mix to-gether plants with a shallow web, a medium root ball, and deep, narrow taproots. Also consider light preferences. Tall sun-loving plants protect shorter shade-loving plants. A bush or tree with lacy leaves can also provide dappled shade under-neath, which many other plants enjoy.

Herbs have qualities that make them good companions. Some have flowers that attract beneficial insects. Others have strong substances to repel pests. A few gather nutrients from the subsoil and bring those within reach of other plants. Here are some herbs that make good neighbors.

Basil discourages flies and mosquitoes. Planted near to-matoes, it enhances their taste. Do not plant near rue.

Bergamot attracts bees, butterflies, and hummingbirds. It improves the growth and flavor of tomatoes.

Borage aids tomatoes by repelling tomato hornworms. Its blue flowers also attract bees. The deep roots bring up valuable nutrients. It makes a good neighbor for squash and strawberries.

Calendula attracts beneficial insects.

Caraway is a miner plant that breaks through and loosens packed or heavy soil. Intersperse it with other plants to help their roots breathe. Caraway also improves the growth and flavor of peas.

Catnip repels ants, flea beetles, and rodents. Plant it as a border to keep them out of a garden.

Chamomile is a "healer" plant. It boosts the immune system and growth of many other plants. It also repels flies and mosquitoes. Use it as a border or in gaps within other plantings.

Chives can protect against aphids, cabbage moths, green flies, mildew, and slugs. They support the health of brassicas, capsicums, carrots, fruit trees, potatoes, roses, and tomatoes. Beneath apple trees, chives prevent apple scab; under roses, they curb blackspot. The pink or white flowers attract bees and butterflies, and occasionally hummingbirds.

Clover fixes nitrogen, providing food for all surrounding plants. Mix white clover into your lawn. Plant red clover along the edges of beds. Leafy herbs such as basil or lettuce use a lot of nitrogen.

Comfrey is a prodigious miner, bringing minerals up to the surface soil, especially potassium. It can be slashed and composted in place several times per growing season. Alternatively, the leaves may be soaked in water to produce a fertilizer tea for foliar feeding. Comfrey supports the health of nearby plants and makes a good garden barrier. The dangling blue flowers attract bees.

Costmary can be made into a tea that kills or repels insect pests when sprayed on foliage.

Dill lures cabbage butterflies away from cabbage. Its flowers attract beneficial insects. It aids the growth of carrots, corn, cucumber, lettuce, and tomatoes.

Elderberry produces a general insecticide. Its leaves aid compost fermentation. Panicles of creamy flowers attract pollinators.

Fennel attracts predatory insects. It repels ants, fleas, and flies. It does not play well with many other plants, so it's best to set it a little way apart.

Feverfew attracts bees and butterflies.

Garlic repels Japanese beetles and many other pests. Plant it near roses to protect them. Garlic also deters herbivores from nibbling or digging in the garden.

Great fleabane is a strong natural insecticide. Use it sparingly and keep it away from beneficial insects.

Horehound deters grasshoppers. It boosts the yield of tomato plants.

Horseradish planted near potatoes will discourage potato bugs and produce more disease-resistant potato tubers.

Hyssop lures cabbage butterflies away from brassicas. Keep it away from radishes.

Lavender has a sharp, soapy smell that confuses pests. It repels mice, rabbits, mosquitoes, moths, and ticks. Bees and butterflies like its blue to purple flower spikes.

Lemon balm supports the health and growth of nearby plants. It also attracts bees. Plant it with cucumbers and tomatoes.

Lovage improves the health and flavor of other plants, especially beans and sweet peppers.

Marigolds repel nematodes, white flies, and other pests. Choose heritage flowers with a strong, sharp smell—many modern varieties have been bred for minimal odor, but the smell comes from the repellant chemicals in the plant. Marigolds also attract hoverflies.

Marjoram attracts beneficial insects. It's a good companion for all herbs and vegetables, especially sage and sweet peppers.

Mint attracts bees with its flowers. It repels cabbage white moths, flies, and mice. Dried, it also protects clothing from moths. Plant mint with cabbage and tomatoes. Contain it carefully so it does not run rampant.

Mustard deters nematodes and some additional root pests.

Nasturtiums attract hoverflies into the garden. These beneficial insects produce larvae that feed on aphids. Nasturtiums bait cabbage white moths. Their strong smell may confuse pests, repelling aphids, cucumber beetles, squash bugs, and striped pumpkin beetles. This is a good companion for cabbage, cucumbers, and radishes. A climbing variety helps apple trees against codling moths. Nasturtiums make an excellent ground cover to trap soil, nutrients, and water. They also serve as a living mulch.

Oregano boosts the growth of beans and other vining plants. It's a good companion to all vegetables. Oregano flowers attract beneficial insects.

Parsley attracts swallowtail butterflies because it is a larval food for them. It also attracts predatory insects that eat pests. Parsley aids the growth and health of other plants near it, especially asparagus, carrots, chives, roses, and tomatoes.

Peppermint attracts bees and discourages pests.

Pyrethrum repels many insect pests. It also produces a potent insecticide; use sparingly and keep away from beneficial insects.

Rosemary has a sharp, piney odor that confuses and repels pests including bean beetles, cabbage moths, and carrot flies. It helps deter dogs and cats from digging. Plant rosemary with sage for mutual support.

Rue has a potent smell that repels many insect pests. It also discourages animals from digging or nibbling in the garden. Its leaves can be used to repel insects, but don't get it on your skin—it can cause contact sun sensitivity. Rue goes well with raspberries and roses, but not with basil, cabbage, or sage.

Sage attracts beneficial insects, especially when flowering. It protects against cabbage white moths. Plant sage with rosemary for mutual support.

Southernwood produces a strong chemical in its leaves that drives away many insect pests, such as cabbage moths. Use it as a border to keep insects from eating the garden.

Summer savory combines favorably with garlic, chives, and other plants in the onion family. With beans, it enhances their flavor and helps protect against bean beetles.

Tansy discourages ants, flies, and moths. Plant some under peach trees to deter flying insect pests. The leaves aid compost fermentation.

Thyme deters cabbageworms and whitefly when planted near cabbage. It also draws bees to tomatoes, potatoes, and eggplant.

Valerian stimulates the growth of all other plants and vegetables nearby. Its pink to white flowers attract butterflies. It also draws in earthworms.

Wormwood produces a strong smell that confuses pests to keep them away from desirable plants. It can be used to make a tea for spraying to control aphids, caterpillars, flea beetles, fleas, flies, and moths. It helps discourage animals from digging in the garden. Grow wormwood in containers or isolated spots, as it can suppress the growth of plants around it. Alternatively, use it as a border to contain aggressive spreaders such as mint.

Yarrow discourages insect pests. It brings up copper, iron, potassium, and sulphur from the subsoil. Plant extra so you can pull some for the compost pile. Yarrow is another "healer" plant that protects and enhances those around it. When flowering, it attracts predatory insects, bees, and butterflies. Yarrow is a good companion for corn, cucumbers, and most herbs. It enhances the development of essential oils.

Attracting Wildlife Partners

Permaculture models human-designed garden space after wilderness. It uses patterns developed and tested by Gaia to create a functional ecosystem in miniature. This includes not just plants but also insects, birds, and other wildlife. They provide pollination, fertilizer, pest control, aesthetic appeal, and more benefits. There is an entire ecosystem in the compost pile alone, known as the detritus food chain.

Remember to use only natural, low-impact pest control so as not to harm your beneficial species. They will keep the pests in check if you provide suitable habitat for them. Provide a mulch pile and wood pile for sheltering insects, amphibians, and birds. Water in a pond or other source attracts all kinds of wildlife. A balanced system creates healthy, vigorous herbs for you to enjoy.

Bees like blue or yellow flowers with a strong scent. Both pollen and nectar appeal to them, and they like bowl-shaped as well as complex flowers. Their favorite herbs include angelica, bergamot, borage, catmint, clover, comfrey, dill, echinacea, feverfew, horehound, lavender, lemon balm, mint, nasturtium, rosemary, sage, savory, sunflower, tansy, thyme, valerian, woad, and yarrow.

Butterflies like large flowers, preferably pink or lavender, with a good landing field. They feed on nectar and prefer scented to unscented flowers. These include bergamot, chives, dill, echinacea, fennel, lavender, rose, verbena, and yarrow. However, butterflies also need larval food plants. Choose from borage, dill, fennel, parsley, and rue.

Birds don't care about scent. Hummingbirds love red tubular flowers full of nectar, such as mallow, pineapple sage, or red bergamot. Seed-eating birds enjoy anything that produces copious edible seeds, such as echinacea, marigold, milk thistle, sunflower, or yarrow. Fruit-eating birds enjoy fruiting herbs, like blackberry, elderberry, mulberry, raspberry, strawberry, and wild cherry.

Herb Garden Design

Permaculture offers several design ideas that work well for herbs. A guild is any group of plants that work together for mutual benefit; there are guilds of edible and medicinal herbs built around fruit or nut trees, for example. A keyhole garden may have a horseshoe shape, or several connected keyholes may form a mandala. An herb spiral combines many plants in a compact, upright space. Pocket plantings nestle herbs into the landscape as a whole rather than containing them in a separate garden.

A guild has layers of plants above and below ground, occupying different niches in the sun and root zones. These span trees, shrubs, vines, herbs, ground covers, and root plants. A tree or shrub provides shelter, scaffolding, shade, and often some kind of nut or fruit. Herbaceous plants produce nitrogen, nutrients, mulch, pollination, and protection along with useful leaves or roots. A nut guild might feature an oak tree, a redbud tree, several white currant bushes, wormwood, yarrow, and woodland strawberries. A fruit guild might include an apple tree with daffodils around the trunk and a dripline border of chives, enclosing a community of asparagus, clover, echinacea, feverfew, mint, oregano, and a rosebush. Gardeners with plentiful space may choose one or more complete guilds.

A keyhole garden is a raised bed protected with mulch, usually in the shape of a horseshoe, with the open end pointed toward the sun (south, in the Northern Hemisphere). Everything can be reached from the central path, creating an efficient use of space. Shorter plants go on the inside, taller ones around the outside. One example uses an inner border of basil and garlic chives, then a row of tomatoes interplanted with marigolds, and finally sunflowers around the outside. In a small yard, the horseshoe is optimal. With more space, chain them together into a keyhole border or mandala garden.

An herb spiral is a specialized rock garden with a concise planting plan. The center of the garden is elevated by means of a coiled rock wall. Plants that love dry, sunny conditions go at the top. Those that favor moderate conditions are found along the sides of the spiral. The base lets out into a small pond for growing watercress and other herbs that need wet or moist habitat. Top: aloe, rosemary, sage. Dry upper area: echinacea, oregano, tarragon, yarrow. Middle: basil, borage, cilantro, parsley. Wet bottom area: miniature cattail, mint, sweet flag, watercress. Tuck creepers, such as creeping thyme and pennyroyal, into niches between the rocks. You may want to shade one side with a woody herb such as bay laurel, elderberry, or rose planted just outside the border.

Pocket plantings include small beds as well as individual plants tucked wherever they will fit. Use these to fill niches in a larger plan. Some good choices include asparagus, clover, garlic, ginger, horseradish, lavender, mint, raspberry, rhubarb, and strawberry.

Elizabeth Barrette *has been involved with the Pagan community for more than twenty-four years. She served as Managing Editor of* PanGaia *for eight years and Dean of Studies at the Grey School of Wizardry for four years. She has written columns on beginning and intermediate Pagan practice, Pagan culture, and Pagan leadership. Her book* Composing Magic: How to Create Magical Spells, Rituals, Blessings, Chants, and Prayers *explains how to combine writing and spirituality. She lives in central Illinois, where she has done much networking with Pagans in her area, such as coffeehouse meetings and open sabbats. Her other public activities feature Pagan picnics and science fiction conventions. She enjoys magical crafts, historic religions, and gardening for wildlife. Her other writing fields include speculative fiction, gender studies, and social and environmental issues. Visit her blog* The Wordsmith's Forge, *http://ysabetwordsmith.livejournal .com, or her website* PenUltimate Productions, *http://penultimate productions.weebly.com. Her coven site with extensive Pagan materials is* Greenhaven Tradition, *http://greenhaventradition.weebly.com.*

Blessed Bees

᭙ By Susan Pesznecker ᭙

M ost of us have a rather complicated relationship with bees.
As small children, we begin with an
innocent fascination, delighting in
watching the insects fly from flower
to flower, watching the dip and sway
of their movements and maybe
even hearing their low hum. We're
delighted, that is, until we receive
our first sting and with it, our loss of
innocence. Or perhaps, if we avoid
being stung, we become aware of
others' fear of bees as they shriek and
swat and run. However it happens,
we come to feel that we can't trust
these well-meaning little creatures. A
lifetime of fear and skepticism is born.

Perhaps this is what makes people today treat bees as if they are not

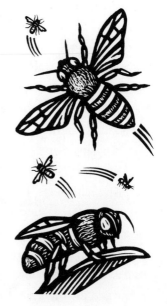

only objects of fear but also unworthy of respect. In either case, we've got it wrong. Not only are bees friendly, civilized, and absolutely fascinating, but as our chief pollinators they are integral to our lives on Earth. And this is critical because bees today are under siege from colony collapse disorder. Bees are in trouble, and if we don't help them find safe ground, we'll be in trouble, too.

All about Bees

Let's start by talking about what we mean by the word "bee," which gets loosely tossed around to describe both bees and wasps. What's the difference? Both bees and wasps belong to the order Hymenoptera, from a Greek root meaning "membraned wings." If you've ever really looked closely at a bee, you'll know exactly what this means, for their wings are transparent and gossamer in appearance. Bees (genus *Apidae*) are small flying insects that produce honey and beeswax and play a critical role in pollinating flowering plants. Honeybees and bumblebees are examples of the bee family. Wasps (family Vespidae) are also small flying insects, but they do not assist with pollination (other than inadvertently), they're carnivorous, and they either prey on or parasitize other insects, arachnids, and even small animals. Well-known wasps include yellow jackets and hornets. For the purposes of this article, we'll focus on bees and particularly on the honeybee.

Like all insects, bees have a three-segmented body (head, abdomen, thorax) and six legs, in addition to their paired wings. Bees also have long, coiled tongues, allowing them to extract nectar from flowers. Bumblebees—the fuzzy, teddy-bear bees that buzz and bumble around flowers—also have specialized *corbiculae* on their hind legs, modifications allowing them to gather "bushels" (on a bee scale) of pollen as they move from flower to flower. If you've watched bumblebees working and have seen yellow "lumps" on their hind legs, you've seen those little corbiculae bushels, full of collected pollen.

Different species of honeybees and bumblebees can be found all over the world, with the exception of the cold polar regions. For the most part, if you look around you and see plants growing, you'll find bees close by. While there are as many as twenty thousand species of bees, the European honeybee is what we think of as the "classic" honeybee—the little fuzzy golden guy we watch happily working over a bed of flowers.

Should We Be Afraid?

Of honeybees? Absolutely not. The only way these little guys will sting you is if they have no other choice, and that usually means you've accidentally grabbed or stepped on one. The result for you is a painful sting, but the result is even worse for the honeybee: his stinger is attached to his innards, and once he buries his stinger in something or someone, his guts are pulled out along with it. Poor bee…

But fear? Nope. Honeybees are incredibly docile, which is why beekeepers are so easily able to collect and work with hives, moving bees from place to place and taking honey from the hives without too much trouble. I have a bank of lavender in my yard, and at summer's peak, the bushes will literally be humming with happy bee action. Those little honeybees are so completely lost in the lavender haze that I can pet them very gently with my fingertips and they don't even seem to notice me.

Now, wasps? That's another story. Wasps are carnivorous and aggressive, and if a wasp is angered or irritated, it may give chase and attack. Wasps also may attack spontaneously if there is potential food nearby and they sense a threat or a challenge. We've all had the experience of enjoying an outdoor picnic and suddenly having yellow jackets appear and begin dive-bombing our food. Many people just abandon their plates, while others start jumping around and swatting at the wasps. Swatting is never a good idea, and it's probably the quickest way to be stung. However, I've also heard others say, "If you hold still, you won't be stung," only to have wasps spontaneously dive-bomb and sting them seconds later. The best advice I can give you? Humans and wasps don't go well together. If you're eating outdoors in a yellow-jackety area, keep your food covered. One successful approach is to make the wasps their own plate, with a piece of meat or fish and a nice bit of ripe fruit. Set the plate a distance away from the humans; it won't take long at all before they'll find this "easy" food, and with any luck they'll leave the rest of your party alone.

What if you're stung? Honeybees leave a stinger behind. Don't squeeze it, for that pushes more venom into the skin. Instead, flick it off with the edge of a pocketknife or credit card. Wasps don't leave a stinger—in fact, one wasp can sting repeatedly. Applying cold packs will relieve pain, and some folks swear by a paste made of mud, baking soda, or meat tenderizer and applied to the sting. Topical cortisone and anti-itch creams will help, too, as will an oral dose of antihistamine (diphenhydramine hydrochloride is ideal). And, of course, you can turn to herbal preparations as remedies: plantain compresses, calendula infusions, and lavender essential oil work quite well.

A small subset of people are violently allergic to bee stings, even to the point that the stings cause a life-threatening condition known as "anaphylactic shock." The greatest danger comes from wasps, but even honeybees can cause serious problems for some people. If you know someone with a dangerous bee allergy, be sure she always has an EpiPen nearby. These devices auto-inject a life-saving dose of epinephrine (adrenaline) that can help stop the allergic reaction. Of course, anyone can become allergic to bees at any time, so if you're with someone who has been stung and suddenly has trouble breathing, develops hives or facial swelling, or is on the verge of collapse, call 9-1-1 and prepare to perform rescue breathing and CPR if indicated.

Bees under Siege

In recent years, beehives and colonies have shown sudden, unexplained episodes of collapse, with tens of thousands of bees suddenly dropping dead. This syndrome has come to be known as colony collapse disorder (CCD) and is the focus of investigation worldwide. Although the cause isn't fully understood, it's believed that neonicotinoid pesticides may be largely to blame. In 2013, near my hometown of Portland, Oregon, fifty thousand honeybees suddenly dropped dead from a grove of trees over the space of an hour, victims of these pesticides. People were so upset and so moved by this, an on-site memorial was held days later for the dead bees.

Most countries are now passing legislation limiting use of these chemicals, and investigation into CCD continues. The world is increasingly aware of the disaster that will result if our bee pollinators continue to be decimated.

How Can We Help the Bees?

First and foremost, educate yourself and others about bees. Too often, people see a bee and haul out the bug spray. This is misguided, because not only does this kill the bee, but the chemicals also damage other plants and animals and often do so in ways we can't always anticipate. As a rule, bees should be welcomed into the yard and respected for their importance to our food chain. Wasps may not be as welcome but should be removed by one's local bee experts. Never knock down a wasp's nest with a rake or a jet of water, and *never* spray it with one of those cans of wasp killer, because seconds later, you'll be under siege by dozens of wasps, who respond to a self-generated chemical DANGER signal and attack en masse.

Second, organic gardening is the bee's best friend, and helping bees means discontinuing the use of chemical fertilizers, herbicides, and insecticides. Many of these are toxic to bees themselves, while others affect the plants that bees use for shelter or food. Even those that do not outright kill the bees can affect them neurologically, making it impossible for the bees to work efficiently or to navigate back to their hives. And, of course, the chemical-affected bee will carry the chemical back to its nest with potentially catastrophic results. Most of these chemicals are also organotoxic, and remain active in the soil with damaging actions for long periods of time before breaking down.

Third, grow plants that attract bees. The plants that bees love most tend to be relatively hardy, gorgeous, and easy to manage. Fruit trees are a wonderful choice for a bee-friendly yard and will yield a crop of fruit to boot. Ditto for berry bushes. Flowers are always an excellent choice, whether as shrubs, plants, or flowering trees. Some bee favorites include lilac, manzanita, calendula (pot marigold), lobelia, columbine, snapdragon, fuchsia, sunflowers, penstemon, and Russian sage.

The honey bees and bumblebees in my yard absolutely adore my flowering herbs, particularly favoring lavender, Echinacea (coneflower), oregano, thyme, and any of the mints. For best results, do some research on bee-favored plants in your region, then have some fun making your bee garden happen.

Fourth, think about bee-friendly landscaping. Bees value shade as well as sun, and they appreciate trees and shrubbery as places to rest and to escape rain, wind, and cold. They may like the convenience, too. In my own yard, I've observed bumble-bees tucking themselves into nearby fir boughs and overnighting there so as to remain close to a bank of flowering lavender. Apparently they wanted to wake up early and be first in line for pollen!

Fifth, bees need water, too. This is especially true in hot climates and in situations where bees must cross large expanses of concrete or asphalt en route back to their nests. These humanmade surfaces retain heat, and bees can easily become overwhelmed by the radiated heat, particularly in hot weather. Provide a water source in your garden: even a terracotta saucer of water, lined with pebbles so the bees don't drown, will be welcomed and might be lifesaving.

Sixth, buy responsibly. Purchase organic honey from ethical beekeepers, and purchase produce that is organic or raised using bee-friendly practices. Doing this helps keeps bee-harming chemicals out of the ecosystem and ensures that your produce and honey have been raised and gathered responsibly and respectfully.

And, of course, if you're able, contribute financially to bee-supporting causes. The Nature Conservancy and the American Beekeeping Federation are doing active work to investigate colony collapse disorder, as are various local, state, and national agencies. A number of companies have also adopted production practices to support the bees, if you'll indulge me, well-bee-ing. Working together, we can help the little guys buzz along indefinitely.

Resources

The New Sunset Western Garden Book. Des Moines, IA: Oxmoor, 2012.

Ransome, Hilda M. *The Sacred Bee in Ancient Times and Folklore*. Mineola, NY: Dover, 2004.

Susan Pesznecker *is a writer, college English teacher, nurse, and hearth Pagan/Druid living in northwestern Oregon. She holds a master's degree in nonfiction writing and loves to read, watch the stars, camp with her wonder poodle, and work in her own biodynamic garden. She is Dean of Students—teaching nature studies and herbology—in the online Grey School of Wizardry (greyschool. com). Sue has authored* The Magickal Retreat *(Llewellyn 2012),* Crafting Magick with Pen and Ink *(Llewellyn, 2009), and* Gargoyles *(New Page, 2007). Visit her on her web page (www.susan pesznecker.com) and her Facebook author page (www.facebook.com /SusanMoonwriterPesznecker).*

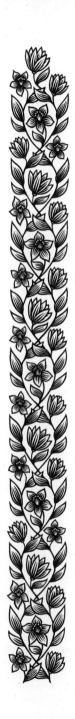

Culinary
Herbs

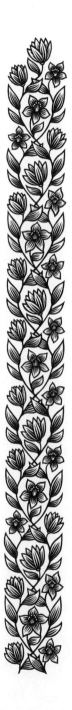

Delightful Dill

≫ By Ember Grant ≪

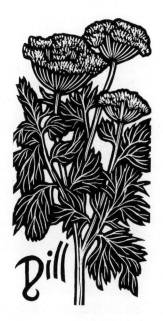

Say the word "dill" and many people immediately think of pickles,
but the herb has so much more to
offer. Adding this graceful plant to
your garden is good for you and the
environment. Dill is one of the easiest
herbs to grow and one of the tastiest
to eat.

Like most herbs we enjoy today,
dill has a long history. The first recorded use of it can be traced back
to the Egyptians nearly five thousand
years ago. The Greeks and Romans
used dill as well—for seasoning, to
preserve vegetables, and for its fragrance. Folklore suggests that dill was
used paradoxically to repel works of

magic and also to create magic. It was especially favored for use in love potions. Since dill was considered an aphrodisiac, it was often added to wine to increase passion.

But dill may be best known for its medical uses, a list that includes aiding indigestion and stomach ailments, reducing flatulence, stimulating appetite, and quelling nausea. In addition, dill seeds are said to freshen the breath when chewed, and an infusion of dill can help sleeplessness. With its calming properties, dill has a reputation for soothing fussy babies and reducing colic. It's also a remedy for headaches. Dill seeds are mildly sedative; dill tea has been used to treat insomnia. In fact, the name dill comes from the Anglo-Saxon *dylle* and the Norse *dilla*—both mean to "lull" or "soothe." Dill seeds were often eaten during church services to ease hunger, giving them the nickname of Meetin' House seeds or House seeds.

Dill, *Anethum graveolens,* is a cousin to the carrot. It is part of the Apiaceae family, one of the largest families of flowering plants, which also includes anise, parsley, caraway, Queen Anne's lace, fennel, and celery. Dill is sometimes referred to as false fennel due to their similar appearance.

Dill is easy to grow from seed and can be grown in zones 2–9. It loves long, warm summers and needs lots of sunlight. There are many varieties of dill, depending on the strengths desired—seeds or foliage. It reaches heights of three feet and may need to be staked when it gets tall or plants will be easily blown over in the wind. Flowers with yellow, green, or white umbels are produced in summer to fall.

Grow dill in well-drained soil to avoid root rot and don't over-water. Sow seeds two to three weeks apart for a continuous harvest. If you live in an area where dill is grown as an annual, collect some seeds to sow for next season. Trim regularly during the growing season to avoid the plants going to seed before you're ready.

Harvesting is simple—cut the fresh leaves as needed. For the strongest fragrance, pick leaves early in the morning after the dew dries. The fresh leaves last about three days in the refrigerator, but you can make them last longer by placing the stems in a glass of water. For long-term storage, you can easily freeze sprigs of dill by packing the plants in freezer bags and squeezing out the air. Or, if you prefer, dry the leaves on a screen and store them in airtight containers away from bright light. Late in the season, when the seeds are golden brown, cut the seed heads and hang them in paper bags or dry them on paper. In about two weeks, when the heads have dried, you should be able to easily crush them with your fingers to remove the seeds.

Dill makes a great companion for cucumbers in the garden as well as in the kitchen. Dill draws butterflies such as the black swallowtail, which lays eggs on the herb and uses it as a host plant for the larvae. Dill is also a valuable nectar plant and attracts beneficial insects, such as ladybugs, that feed on aphids and other pests.

The main reason most people grow dill is for use in the kitchen. While this herb is native to the Mediterranean region and parts of Asia, the use of dill has spread around the world and is popular in the cuisine of many cultures. The fresh leaves are commonly used in dips and on baked fish, and the seeds are similar in flavor to caraway seed. The leaves can be used fresh or dried, although the flavor is stronger when they're fresh. The dried leaves are sold as dill weed to avoid confusion between the leaves and the seeds.

Dill Recipes and Crafts

Here are some of my favorite dill recipes and crafts. The first recipe has been in my family for more than four generations.

Dilled Cucumbers and Onions

> ½ cup sugar
>
> ½ cup white wine vinegar
>
> 1 white onion
>
> ½ teaspoon white pepper (optional)
>
> 1 tablespoon salt
>
> 1 tablespoon dried dill (dill weed)
>
> 3 cucumbers

Peel and slice the cucumbers thinly. Slice the onion. Mix all the ingredients in a large bowl, cover, and refrigerate overnight. The volume of liquid will increase as the cucumbers soften. This makes a delicious side dish for a summer barbeque and is sometimes called cucumber salad.

Dill Honey

Use 1 tablespoon of fresh, washed dill (and other herbs as desired) for every two cups of honey. Crush the herbs slightly and either place them in a cheesecloth bag or directly into a saucepan. Pour the honey over the herbs and heat until warm but not hot. Next, pour the mixture into a hot, sterilized jar and seal tightly. Store at room temperature for about a week, then rewarm the honey and strain out the herbs or remove the bag. Or you can leave the loose herbs in the honey, if you wish. Return the honey to hot, sterilized jars once again for storage, and seal.

Dill Vinegar and Oils

A delicious herb vinegar can be made using red wine vinegar and dill or a combination of dill and chives. Begin by washing and drying the herbs, then pack them into hot, sterilized jars. Add vinegar, allowing one inch of space at the top. Using a wooden spoon, push the herbs down, bruising them slightly. Cover the jars with plastic before adding the metal lids, then screw tight to seal. Let the mixture steep in a dark place for three to six weeks, then strain using a coffee filter. Pour the vinegar into hot, sterilized jars once again or decorative bottles. Add a few sprigs of fresh herb, if desired, and cap. This makes a great gift and can be used in most recipes that call for vinegar. Try combining different herbs with red or white wine vinegar.

Herbal oils are prepared in much the same way using olive or vegetable oil. Just put the herbs in a hot, sterilized jar and add warmed oil. Let the oil cool, then cover tightly and store in the refrigerator.

Dill Soak and Infusion

Dill is famous for its fragrance, so here are some ways to take advantage of the delightful aroma and pamper yourself in the process. For a relaxing soak, wrap fresh dill in cheesecloth. Tie the bundle tightly and add to your bath. To strengthen fingernails, make an infusion of dill seeds and allow it to cool. Soak fingernails in the mixture for ten minutes. Repeat daily or as needed.

Dill Pillow

Make a dill pillow to aid sleep by sewing the leaves inside fabric. First, cut two squares of your desired size and stitch three of the sides, right sides together. Turn the fabric inside out and stuff with the herbs. Be sure to remove any sharp stems. Stitch the top together and place in your pillowcase.

Tussie-Mussie

Dill is a wonderful addition to fragrant miniature bouquets called tussie-mussies, or nosegays. In medieval times, these were used to disguise offensive odors due to poor sanitation. In addition, the plants included in the bouquets could be interpreted as symbols to send secret messages. In the language of flowers, dill stands for good cheer and persistence.

To make a tussie-mussie, select the herb or flower that you wish to have the most prominence and place it in the center. Surround it with other plants—flowers and herbs with fragrances you enjoy, those in your favorite colors, or those with symbolic meanings.

Secure the stems with a rubber band or floral tape. Cut an X in a paper doily and push the stems through, cupping the flowers and securing the doily in place with more tape if needed. Place the bouquet in a vase of water. Alternately, you can give these as gifts—attach ribbons in various colors and a card to explain what each plant means. These bouquets can even be dried and used to add fragrance to a room.

Dill is one of my favorite herbs in the garden and in the kitchen. Those soft, feathery fronds are beautiful, delicious, and aromatic. It's not harvest time at my home without making my favorite dilled cucumbers—made with my homegrown cucumbers, of course! Once you experience all dill has to offer, you'll want to enjoy it year round.

Bibliography

Michalak, Patricia S. *Rodale's Successful Organic Gardening: Herbs*. Emmaus, PA: Rodale Press, 1993.

Picton, Margaret. *The Book of Magical Herbs: Herbal History, Mystery, and Folklore*. New York: Barron's, 2000.

Webb, Marcus A., and Richard Craze. *The Herb & Spice Companion*. London: Oceana/Quantum Publishing, 2000.

Ember Grant *is the author of two books,* Magical Candle Crafting *and* The Book of Crystal Spells, *and she has been writing for the Llewellyn annuals since 2003. Ember is a college English teacher and also enjoys nature photography and gardening. Visit her online at embergrant.com.*

Signature Sipping: Making Your Own Herbal Tea Blends

≈ By Dallas Jennifer Cobb ≈

Walk into any supermarket or health food store and you will find row upon row and shelf after shelf of herbal teas. Beautiful boxes decorated with bright colors sit side by side bags of loose herbs bearing lovely labels, and nearby are the handcrafted, individually created niche-market teas. There are literally hundreds of herbal combinations ready-made, available in prepared tea bags or loose. Many of these blends are made with taste in mind and bear names that inspire and delight.

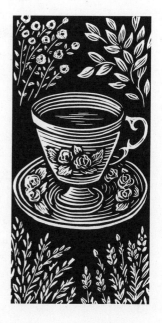

But what if you are not an over-the-counter type of person and would really prefer the practice of making your own signature blend of herbal tea? Maybe you haven't found that perfect blend on the shelf and long to create your own signature sipping brew. Maybe you have a garden and long to learn how to capture the taste of that perfect summer night. Or maybe you have a health issue that can be aided by herbs and want to create your own tasty tea.

Each of us has different needs in a tea, depending on our age, gender, health, lifestyle, and taste preferences. And finding, or inventing, our own "signature" tea is a deeply personal and empowering process.

This article is about making your own particular herbal tea: a personal blend of herbs that are specific to your lifestyle, health, and spiritual needs—a tea that is your signature combination. Now you can enjoy something that was made just for you. And the process of making your own signature sipping blend will allow you to contemplate your personal preferences and design something personally affirming.

Making Perfect Tea

While we think of Canada and the United States as coffee countries, more tea is consumed worldwide than coffee. In fact, tea is the second most popular drink in the world after water. Tea is also known as a tisane or an infusion. Herbal teas are prepared in the same way that black tea is prepared.

Your Signature Sip

When you first decide to make your own signature sipping blend, you might feel overwhelmed and wonder, where do I start? For me, a few simple questions helped to steer me in the right direction.

Decide first, do I want caffeine or no caffeine?

Black, white, and green teas all contain caffeine. In the average eight-ounce cup of black tea, there are up to 60 milligrams of caffeine, whereas green tea contains up to 40 milligrams, white tea up to 25 milligrams, and decaffeinated black tea up to 15 milligrams. Many tasty blends are made with black tea as their basis, such as traditional chai and British flavored teas.

Next ask yourself, what feeling do I want my tea to evoke?

For relaxation, consider using chamomile, lavender, or lemon balm as your flavorful base, and add the healing effects of catnip or vervain. If you want inspiration, use the stimulating flavors of peppermint, lavender, or spearmint, and add calendula, St. John's wort, or lemon balm to brighten your spirits. Is your soul in need of soothing? Use the calming flavor of licorice root with the healing nature of catnip or rosemary.

Is the tea for a man or a woman?

Depending on your gender, you may choose different herbs that have a therapeutic effect on the sexual and reproductive organs of women and men. Common "women's" herbs include alfalfa, Beth root, black cohosh, chaste tree, clary sage, cramp bark, dong quai, epimedium, fennel seed, lady's mantle, maca root, red clover, sage, and wild yam root. Common "men's" herbs include Asian ginseng, gingko biloba, horny goat weed, St. John's wort, and saw palmetto.

What spiritual energy do I need?

When I make my own signature sipping blends, I always consider the spiritual energy of herbs. As a highly vibrating natural substance, herbs impart many gifts, and if you are open to them energetically, they will bless you. Angelica carries a protective and healing energy and promotes creativity and inspiration. The delicate calendula flower instills joy and blesses dreams. Because it follows the sun with its tiny face, much in the same way the majestic sunflower does, calendula is also known for its guardian qualities. Chamomile is for bravery and overcoming challenges. Not only will it settle your stomach, but it can heal bad dreams and promote peace.

If you long to open your heart and experience more success in the world, drink fennel. It will help you to see the deeper spiritual lessons that are at hand. Lavender vibrates with truth and joy. Know that all is well in your life and that the universe supports your growing joyfulness. To relax and release old wounds, drink delicious lemon balm. Let go, let lemon balm, and brightly bounce back spiritually.

Want to enjoy money, prosperity, abundance, and success? Add some peppermint to your signature sip. A stimulant that both uplifts and reignites the internal fire, it will help energize your greater good. Remember rosemary, and open the doors to past-life awareness, the resolution of early life dramas, and greater spiritual understanding. Rosemary can help you align yourself with your deepest dreams. And to focus more on your spiritual goals, turn to thyme, the herbal symbol of magic. It will remind you that magic is the ability to change energy at will, and thyme can easily help to shift many kinds of energy.

What health issues do I need to address?

Ideally, your signature sipping blend takes your health into consideration and includes herbs that aid and promote good health both generally and specific to your concerns. I like to keep it simple, so I am listing here only a few herbs that are commonly grown throughout North America and are readily available in grocery and health food stores. Each of these herbs is also quite versatile and can be combined in a variety of ways with many other herbs.

Catnip (*Nepeta cataria*) is part of the mint family and has a lovely earthy, mint flavor. It reduces fevers, calms the nervous system, and eases insomnia.

Chamomile (*Chamaemelum nobile*) is a sweet-tasting, mild flower. It produces a gorgeous golden hue in the water and possesses calming qualities. It is often used to relieve upset stomachs, ease teething pains, and calm colic, insomnia, and nervousness, plus it releases gas.

Lavender (*Lavandula augustifolia*) relieves headaches, eases nervous conditions, and promotes calm. The aromatic purple flowers give tea a hint of blue and produce intoxicating aromas.

Lemon balm (*Melissa officinalis*) has a strong lemon flavor that mixes well with fruity and minty blends. Known for its efficacy in relieving headaches, insomnia, and depression, lemon balm is a wonderful herb to include in your signature sip.

Mint (*Mentha*) comes in so many varieties that many gardens have a few different flavors growing, the most common being *Mentha piperita* (peppermint) and *Mentha spicata* (spearmint). All of the mints are known for relieving nausea and aiding in digestion.

Pot marigold (*Calendula officinalis*) is a lovely orange flower. When dried, it visually brightens up any tea mixture and turns the tea a lovely orange color. Pot marigold is known for its "brightening" qualities, aiding in the relief of depression.

Rosemary (*Rosmarinus officinalis*) is a versatile, savory herb that is widely used in herbal teas. Touted for its effective treatment of poor circulation, indigestion, and even nervous conditions, rosemary has a taste that stimulates memory.

Sage (*Salvia offinalis*) is another versatile herb that should be included in a tea garden. It has been used to coat a sore throat, to gargle away tonsillitis, and to relieve coughs.

Thyme (*Thymus vulgaris*) is a remedy for colds, indigestion, and even asthma. With its delightful flavor, it can be included in many individualized signature sipping teas.

If you suffer from a digestive disorder, consider including any one of the mint family herbs—such as rosemary, thyme, lemon balm, or fennel—as all can aid digestion, relieve stomach upset, and dispel gas. For the common cold or respiratory disorders, consider including rosemary, sage, thyme, or lemon balm in your sipping blend.

Making Marvelous Tea

Herbal tea is easy to make. The "secrets" to know in advance are: always use boiling water, because the heat is what releases the essential oils in the herbs and brings out the particular flavors and gives you access to the active healing qualities; and never use a metal teapot because it changes the taste of the herbs. I prefer a crockery or clay teapot, and find that the "brown betty" style—a thick, round-bodied teapot—keeps tea warmer longer.

Take a clean teapot and rinse it with boiling water to heat it up, so that it retains the heat for a longer period of time. Place fresh or dried herbs in the pot, keeping in mind that it takes almost three times the amount of fresh herbs to achieve the same great taste that you can get from dried herbs. When using dried herbs, I suggest using approximately one teaspoon of herbs per cup of tea, placing the herbs directly into the cup. If you are making a pot, the measurement is a teaspoon per cup, plus one teaspoon "for the pot."

Unless you are going to be doing divination through "tea cup reading" and you specifically want tea leaves in your cup, I recommend using a tea egg (tea ball). Most people don't like having fiber, or bits of herb leaf, in their tea. If your pot has its own internal strainer adjacent to the spout, you might be tempted to put the herbs directly in the pot, but this makes it difficult to take the herbs out to control strength and flavor. The tea egg, a stainless-steel egg-shaped contraption that the herbs are placed in, is filled and placed in the pot. Boiling water is then poured over and through it, and if you are like me, you can hold the chain and dip the egg up and down impatiently.

Pour the boiling water over the herbs and let them steep for five minutes. Even herbal teas will color the water, and once you see the color start to change, the flavor will change, too. After five minutes, strain out or remove the herbs. I don't like to steep longer than five minutes because many herbs grow bitter the longer they are immersed, and I am not a fan of bitter tea. If you like strong tea, then use more herbs from the outset. Strong tea is flavorful, but bitter tea is just bitter.

Once your tea is steeped, serve while the tea is hot. Again, temperature is part of perfect flavor.

Many people enjoy sweetening herbal tea with sugar or honey, but lately I have become a fan of stevia (*Stevia rebaudiana*), a leafy plant with a wonderfully sweet taste. I have started to combine it with other herbs that benefit from a slightly sweet, enhancing flavor. Stevia provides the taste of sweetness without the calories or sugar spike.

Signature Sipping

If you are like me, you won't stop with just one signature sip. I have made a number of my own herbal blends, each with a unique name, including "Dash Away Darkness," "Wake Up and Live Now," and "Lush Hush."

Recently, I started to make signature sipping blends as gifts for my friends. First, I meditate on the person, thinking about his or her personality, character, lifestyle, and health, and then get to work pairing the herbs.

I make up names for their signature sipping blends and enjoy their delight when they open up their own individualized bag of herbal tea. After I have developed the recipe for their tea, I label the blend with its name, the ingredients used, and the date it was made. I adore alliteration and try to find a name that says whom it is for and what it does, such as "Donna's Delicate Delight," "Mom's Majestic Magic," "Sweet Cecelia's Treat," and "Sweet Sipping."

Dallas Jennifer Cobb *practices gratitude magic, giving thanks for personal happiness, health, and prosperity; meaningful, rewarding, and flexible work; and a deliciously joyful life. She is accomplishing her deepest desires. She lives in paradise with her daughter in a waterfront village in rural Ontario, where she regularly swims and runs, chanting: "Thank you, thank you, thank you." Contact her at jennifer.cobb@live.com.*

One-Dish Wonders for a Savory Main Course

≫ By Alice DeVille ≪

Creative cooks and home entertainers learn early in the game that they win raves from guests by creating meals that are easy on the eyes and satisfying to the taste buds. These recipes cover the bases for meat, fish, or poultry lovers as well as diners looking for meatless entrées.

Breakfast or Brunch Specialties

Who doesn't love an invitation to brunch? The host usually offers an array of treats along with a guest-pleasing main course. If you are looking for a savory centerpiece for your next gathering, include this lovely, rich frittata among the possibilities. Why not make two, if expecting a

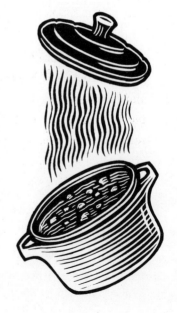

large group, and arrange them on opposite sides of your serving table? Preparation is a snap and it is lip-smacking good, even though a medium slice is close to five hundred calories. You can substitute 3 tablespoons olive oil for the butter and use low-fat cheeses to cut calories, but the taste and consistency may not be as satisfying. This recipe serves 8.

Potato Frittata with Chives

> 1 pound potatoes, peeled and cut into ½-inch cubes
> (2 cups)
>
> 1 stick unsalted butter, melted
>
> ¾ teaspoon salt, divided
>
> ⅓ cup all-purpose flour
>
> ¼ cup chopped fresh chives
>
> ¾ teaspoon baking powder
>
> ½ teaspoon black pepper
>
> 1 15-ounce container of whole milk ricotta cheese
> (or use part-skim)
>
> 12 ounces sharp cheddar cheese, grated
>
> 8 extra-large eggs

Peel and dice potatoes and sauté in the butter in a 10-inch oven-proof or cast iron skillet. Sprinkle with half the salt and cook until potatoes are fork-tender but not falling apart. If your skillet is not ovenproof, wrap the handle in foil.

Preheat oven to 350°F and arrange rack in center of the oven. Whisk together the flour, chopped chives, baking powder, black pepper, and the remaining salt. In another bowl, whisk the cheeses and eggs together until well combined. Then whisk in the flour mixture.

Pour egg mixture over the potatoes in the skillet and bake until firm and puffy, about 45 minutes. Remove from oven and let cool 5–10 minutes. Run a small knife around the edge of the frittata and gently slide onto a platter. Serve warm. Delish!

When you have overnight houseguests or simply want to please your family, this easy-to-prepare baked breakfast treat wins raves. The dish is a tasty, appetizing way to conquer those morning hunger cravings. I use pork sausage in my version, which provides eight generous portions. You can easily substitute with chicken or turkey sausage and follow the instructions. Serve with sweet rolls, toast, butter, and fruit to complement the meal.

Herbed Sweet Sausage Casserole

1 pound bulk sausage, browned and drained

¼ teaspoon ground sage

¼ teaspoon fennel seeds

Nonstick cooking spray or 1 tablespoon solid shortening

4 slices whole grain, challah, or white bread

6 large eggs

2 cups milk (whole preferred)

1 tablespoon yellow or Dijon mustard

½ teaspoon salt

¼ teaspoon fresh ground black pepper

5 ounces grated sharp cheddar cheese

Brown sausage in skillet, breaking up clumps. Add sage and fennel to mixture and stir. After sausage cooks, drain and set aside to incorporate into casserole.

While sausage is browning, preheat oven to 350°F. Coat a 9 × 12-inch baking dish or oval casserole with the cooking spray or evenly coat with solid shortening.

Tear bread of choice into bite-size pieces and scatter over the bottom of the greased dish. Top with cooked sausage.

Use medium bowl to whisk eggs until combined. Whisk in milk, mustard, salt, and pepper. Pour over bread and sausage. Sprinkle cheese over top.

Bake uncovered on middle oven rack for 35–45 minutes or until set all the way to center (insert knife into center until it comes out clean). Let sit for 5 minutes and serve.

A "Wow" Factor Lunch

Entertaining at lunch with this elegant pie gets raves. It's a beauty! I also call it "the one that got away"—I lost it for a while in the Great Divide (a divorce several years ago) and could not get it back. I missed making the dish and sat down one day writing down everything I could remember about it and adding more ingredients. Then I made it and tasted it, and here it is for your enjoyment. Add rolls and salad greens, and dig in to a midday feast.

Elegant Spinach Pie

   3 strips cooked bacon, diced

   1 medium onion, chopped

   1 package frozen chopped spinach, thawed and
      squeezed dry

   1 deep-dish baked pie shell (ready-made or your own
      pie crust)

   4 eggs, slightly beaten

2 cups grated Swiss or Gruyere (sometimes I use a cup
   of each)

1 cup heavy cream

½ teaspoon herbes de Provence

1 teaspoon salt

¼ teaspoon ground black pepper

1 pinch nutmeg

Cook bacon in skillet, then sauté onion with bacon and drain any fat. Add thawed and drained spinach and combine well.

Fill baked pie shell with spinach/bacon/onion mixture.

Combine eggs and cheese, then stir in cream and add the herbes de Provence, salt, pepper, and nutmeg until combined. Pour mixture into pie shell over spinach mixture.

Bake for 20 minutes at 425°F. Then lower temperature to 350°F and bake for an additional 40 minutes until done. Check to make sure crust does not brown too quickly, and cover edges with foil. Poke center with cake tester; if tester comes out clean, your pie is done. Cool for 10 minutes after baking and serve.

A Salad Star

For over thirty years, I have prepared variations of this taco salad recipe, a dish that pleases a crowd at parties as a side dish or works as your main course at lunch or dinner. Ground beef is the star ingredient, or substitute with boneless, skinless chicken breasts or 1 ½ pounds of chicken tenders. You'll need a big wide-rimmed serving platter with plenty of room to mix the ingredients. Cut the recipe in half if you are feeding fewer people and don't want a lot of leftovers, because this recipe makes a lot. The only accompaniments you need are some fresh guacamole (easy recipe follows) and sour cream.

Tempting Taco Salad

- 1 ½ pounds ground beef (or 3 boneless, skinless chicken breasts or 1 ½ pounds of chicken tenders, cubed ½ inch)
- 1 large onion, chopped
- 2 teaspoons each of salt, pepper, and garlic powder
- 2 cans pork and beans or vegetarian baked beans (or your own recipe)
- 1–2 heads lettuce of your choice, shredded
- 2–3 large tomatoes, chopped
- ¼ cup finely grated onion
- 1 pound grated sharp cheddar cheese
- ½ to ¾ bottle of Catalina or French dressing
- 1–2 tablespoons picante sauce (optional)
- 1 bag nacho cheese–flavored Doritos, crushed

Brown beef (or chicken) with chopped onion, salt, pepper, and garlic powder. Add beans and simmer 10 minutes.

Mix lettuce, tomatoes, finely grated onion, and cheese in a large serving platter. Pour beef or chicken mixture over salad. Mix in salad dressing with or without picante, and combine well. Just before serving, add crushed Doritos and stir into mixture.

Easy Guacamole

- 2 ripe avocados, mashed but a little chunky
- 1 crushed garlic clove
- ¼ cup finely minced onion
- ½ teaspoon salt

¼ teaspoon black pepper

1–2 tablespoons squeezed lemon juice

Peel, seed, and mash 2 ripe avocados in medium-size bowl. Add crushed garlic, minced onion, salt, and pepper. Add lemon juice and combine.

Dinner Divine

Everyone seems to have a favorite chicken noodle dish. Most are baked as casseroles, but here's one you can make on your range. Although I serve this tasty creation mostly for dinner, it also makes a wonderful meal when I invite friends over for a leisurely lunch. My real-estate colleagues couldn't resist going for second helpings. All you need is a simple salad and savory bread, and you're ready to feast. The dish brings an all-season aura of palate satisfaction and takes less than an hour to prepare with ingredients you have on hand. Makes 4 servings; double the amount for additional guests.

Lemon-Zested Chicken and Egg Noodles

8 ounces wide egg noodles

½ bag stringless sugar snap peas (8 ounces)

1 cup shredded carrots (packaged or shred your own)

1 cup frozen peas

1 cup chicken broth

½ cup heavy or whipping cream

1 tablespoon grated fresh lemon peel or zest

½ teaspoon coarsely ground black pepper

½–¾ teaspoon salt

2 cups cooked chicken cut in ½-inch pieces
   (use rotisserie chicken to save time)

1 tablespoon chopped flat leaf parsley

½ cup grated sharp cheddar cheese (optional)

Heat a 4-quart covered saucepan of well-salted water to boiling over high heat. Add noodles and cook as label directs, adding snap peas to the noodles about 2 minutes before the noodles are done.

Meanwhile, place carrots and frozen peas in a large colander over the sink. Drain the noodles and snap peas over the carrots and frozen peas so they "cook."

Let the noodle mixture drain, and use the same large saucepan to heat broth, cream, lemon peel, pepper, and salt to boiling over high heat.

Stir the chicken and the noodle mixture into the sauce. Heat thoroughly, stirring constantly. Pour into serving bowl and top with cheddar cheese and chopped parsley. Lip-smacking good!

This dish is my hands-down favorite roast beef meal any time of year. I adapted it from a 1982 *Sunset Easy Basics for Good Cooking* recipe. You can use most boneless cuts of beef, such as rump, sirloin, or chuck roast. My personal preference is an eye of round roast for melt-in-your-mouth tenderness. Depending on the size of your roast, you can easily serve 8 people.

Savory One-Pot Roast Beef

   All-purpose flour for dredging and gravy

   4 to 5-pound boneless roast beef

   2 tablespoons canola or vegetable oil

6 tablespoons butter, divided

1 bay leaf

1 teaspoon ground black pepper

1 ½ teaspoons thyme leaves

1 can (14 ½ ounces) beef broth and 1 ½ cans water

1 teaspoon Kitchen Bouquet

½ cup red wine (optional)

2 onions, peeled and cut into eighths (or 12 white boiling onions, peeled)

4 medium carrots, peeled and cut into 2-inch pieces (or use half a bag of ready-peeled carrots)

3 medium potatoes, peeled and cut into 6 pieces each

4 tablespoons all-purpose flour

Kosher salt (about a teaspoon)

Rub flour into roast, and brush off excess. Heat oil in 5-quart Dutch oven with 2 tablespoons butter over medium heat. Add meat and brown well on all sides. Add bay leaf, pepper, thyme, beef broth, water, Kitchen Bouquet, and red wine, and bring to a boil. Cover and place in a 350°F oven for 1 ½ hours.

Add onions, carrots, and potatoes. Sprinkle lightly with kosher salt. Continue to cook, covered, for 1 ½ hours until roast and vegetables are tender when pierced lightly with a fork.

Transfer roast and vegetables to a rimmed platter, and keep warm with loosely tented foil—do not steam. Skim fat from drippings. Pour drippings into a 4-cup glass measuring cup and add water, if necessary, to make 4 cups total. Carve roast and keep warm while you prepare the gravy. If you like to serve leftovers later in the week and want more gravy on hand, just add another cup of water, 1 tablespoon butter, and 1 more tablespoon flour, and follow above instructions.

Melt the remaining 4 tablespoons butter in Dutch oven over medium heat. Add the 4 tablespoons flour. Add salt to taste and cook, stirring, until bubbly. Remove from heat. With a wire whisk, gradually stir in reserved drippings, then remove bay leaf. Return pan to heat and cook, stirring until thickened. Pour into a gravy boat to pass at the table.

Inspiration for this salmon recipe came from a chance conversation. About ten years ago, I had contractors working on my home. One of them noted that I always had some tantalizing food smells coming from my kitchen and told me he used to be a cook at a notable area restaurant. I asked him about his favorite dish from the eatery, and he told me it was a spicy scalloped salmon dish. He could not remember the details of the mix that coated the salmon, just that it contained cumin, cayenne, salt, garlic powder, and a few other ingredients and could be made with a sauce to serve over pasta. So, Jimmy, wherever you are, here is what I came up with to create a spicy recipe that serves 6–8 people.

Succulent Scalloped Salmon

> 4 six-ounce skinless salmon fillets, sliced into scallops no more than ½-inch thick
>
> Spice mixture to coat salmon (recipe follows)
>
> 1 stick butter, plus 1 tablespoon for sautéing salmon
>
> Juice of 1 large lemon (or 1 cup heavy cream)
>
> 1 teaspoon capers, drained

1 pound thin spaghetti or angel hair pasta

½–¾ cup pasta cooking water, reserved

1 tablespoon canola oil

1–2 tablespoons chopped Italian flat leaf parsley

If using fresh salmon, place the fillets in the freezer for 20 minutes before slicing; they will make a nice clean cut, or scallop, that cooks quickly and absorbs the seasoning and sauce. Prepare the spice mixture (recipe follows).

Meanwhile, decide whether you want a butter-lemon or a cream sauce for your salmon and pasta entrée. Take a 1-quart saucepan and melt the stick of butter over medium-low heat. Add the juice of 1 large lemon and combine. When sauce is heated through, add the teaspoon of capers and set aside.

If you prefer the cream sauce with your salmon, melt the butter in a 1-quart saucepan, then add heavy cream. Add capers when heated through, and set aside to combine with pasta and salmon mixture.

Bring well-salted pasta water to a boil over high heat. Cook pasta of choice according to package directions and drain, reserving ½–¾ cup of pasta water.

In heavy skillet, heat oil and 1 tablespoon butter. When pan is hot, add scalloped salmon and sprinkle generously to taste with spicy seasoning. It is hot, so don't add too much of the seasoning. I use a tablespoon and test for "heat" when salmon is almost done. Be careful not to burn your gums. The salmon will cook in 5–7 minutes. When done, set aside and add to drained pasta in a large pasta serving bowl, then add the sauce mixture and combine. Add the reserved pasta water, combine, and sprinkle with parsley. Ready to serve!

Spicy Seasoning

- 1 ½ tablespoons cumin
- 2 tablespoons granulated garlic
- 2 tablespoons onion powder
- 1 tablespoon paprika
- 1 ½ teaspoons cayenne pepper
- 1 teaspoon black pepper
- 1 ½ tablespoons iodized salt

Combine all ingredients in medium bowl, and store in airtight container away from heat or in refrigerator for up to 6 months. This mix works well with fish, seafood, meat, and poultry. Use in accordance with your personal palate preference.

Sources

Recipes in this article are from the personal handwritten notes and recipe files of Alice DeVille.

Alice DeVille *is an internationally known astrologer, writer, and metaphysical consultant specializing in relationships, health, real estate, government affairs, career and change management, and spiritual development. An accomplished cook, Alice prepares food from a variety of cuisines and enjoys creating new recipes, hosting parties, and organizing holiday feasts. Alice is available for writing books and articles for publishers, newspapers, or magazines and conducting workshops, lectures, and radio or TV interviews. Contact her at DeVilleAA@aol.com or on Twitter @AstroOnDemand, and visit her website at www.astrologyondemand.com.*

Mint: Quite Possibly the World's Most Popular Herb

By Anne Sala

Open your medicine cabinet and count how many mint-flavored products you see. Probably several, right? Mint is perhaps the most recognizable scent in the world. Aside from lavender and rose, there are few scents as familiar or versatile. The smell of mint assures us that our breath is fresh, our hands are clean, and the surfaces we are touching are sanitized.

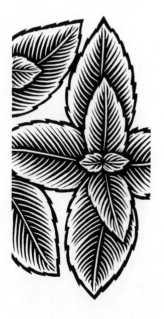

Mint's popularity stems from the menthol oil produced in its leaves. Native to the Mediterranean and Western Asia, mint has been used by humans for thousands of years. It was used in funerary rights, to prevent hangovers, to increase the libido, and to preserve food. The Bible describes the Pharisees being paid tithes of mint and rue. The Romans carried it in their prolific herb arsenal as they settled their empire. To this day, offering mint tea to a guest is considered the most fundamental gesture of hospitality in many cultures.

The two most popular members of the *Mentha* genus are spearmint (*Mentha spicata*) and peppermint (*Mentha piperita*), both of which harbor the purest essence of what "mint should smell like." Through this herb's fondness for hybridization, however, mint's fragrance can also carry a hint of apple, ginger, lemon, and even chocolate. Currently, there are about eighteen different species of mint in the Lamiaceae (or Labiatae) family.

The look of mint is slightly different with each variety. The stems can grow tall or creep along the ground. The paired leaves can be crinkly, round, or ovoid in shape, and come in a range of green hues. At the end of summer, spikes of purple or white flowers form at the tops of the branches, which then turn into seedpods.

Mint's roots are tenacious and put out runners that easily grow new plants. For this reason, mint is often classified as an invasive plant. However, these "volunteer" mints are usually hardier than the plants that come from the seeds, so they are the best way to propagate the herb—or even root the leftover cuttings you buy at the supermarket. Plant them in moist, fertile soil. While most mints will do just fine in full sun, those planted in the shade are thought to have the strongest flavor and scent.

The name "mint" comes from the Greek *mintha*. It is said that the herb is named after a Naiad, or water nymph, who came to a tragic end. Apparently, Minthe had an affair with Hades, the god of the underworld. When his wife, Persephone, found out, she began to savagely kick Minthe, beating her into the ground. While Hades could not prevent his wife from exacting her punishment upon the nymph, he was able to transform his mistress into a plant with a beguiling fragrance.

Another blessing bestowed upon Minthe is how uncomplicated it is to dry her leaves and store them for use year round. Pennyroyal (*Menthe pulegium*) is the preferred variety in the medicine world due to its particularly pungent menthol aroma. This volatile oil imparts a cooling effect, which can relax muscles as well as ease headaches and soothe upset stomachs, though it should not be used by pregnant women. The oils also have antiviral and antioxidant properties. No matter what variety of mint you use, the menthol's scent actually seems to get stronger upon drying.

Mint Recipes

Here is a sampling of recipes that incorporate "the good herb," as it is known in South America. I chose dishes that require mint to truly affect the flavor of the fare, and where mint does not just appear as a sprinkled garnish. That is not to diminish its use as a garnish! Stir it into your lemonade. Pluck the flowers, remove the green bit, and sprinkle on your salad or mix into your rice. I also encourage you to go the traditional route and pair it with lamb, new potatoes, and peas. If nothing else, the scent of mint in your supper will raise your spirits.

I used spearmint in all the recipes because it is the easiest type to find in most markets, but I encourage you to experiment with any variety that you like.

Cucumber Mint Cooler

Drink this when temperatures spike. The freshness of the mint shines through. For a more intense beverage, forgo the soda water and drink the strained purée over ice. Serves 4.

    1 pound Persian cucumbers, cut into chunks

    2 limes, 1 ½ juiced and ½ thinly sliced

    1 ½ cups mint, lightly packed, woody stems removed,
      and more for garnish

    ⅛ cup sugar or to taste

    1–2 cups water

    Ice cubes

    Soda water

Place all the ingredients except for lime slices, mint garnish, and soda water in a blender or food processor. Purée until only small flecks of mint and cucumber peel are visible.

Pour the purée through a fine sieve into a pitcher. Press on the solids with a rubber spatula to expel as much liquid as possible. Discard the solids.

Serve by filling four glasses with ice. Pour in a portion of the cooler and top off with soda water. Garnish with mint and lime. Add a splash of rum, gin, or vodka if you are so inclined.

Raspberry Ginger Mint Iced Tea

When a recipe calls for pouring hot water over mint leaves, I find that the mint flavor remains cleaner when the leaves are dried. The baking soda helps the raspberries retain their color, but it does not affect the flavor. Also, you are welcome to strain out the raspberries at the end of the steeping period, but I like to keep them in for aesthetic reasons. Technically, this is a tisane, but that is too much of a mouthful to say on a hot day. Makes 6 cups.

> 1 thumb-sized piece ginger, peeled
>
> ½ cup fresh raspberries, rinsed
>
> 4 ounces dried mint leaves, or 4 tea bags of mint herbal tea
>
> 2 tablespoons sugar, honey, or simple syrup, or to taste
>
> ⅛ teaspoon baking soda
>
> 6 cups water, divided

Place 4 cups water and ginger in a pan and bring to a rolling boil.

Pour the ginger water into a nonreactive, heat-resistant container and add the rest of the ingredients, except for the additional water. Let steep for 5–10 minutes.

Remove the ginger piece. Add 2 cups cold water, and place in the refrigerator to cool until ready to serve.

Grilled Halloumi and Melon Salad with Mint Vinaigrette

Halloumi is a cheese from Cyprus that does not melt when heated. Instead, the exterior browns and becomes crisp. The secret to this property is the hour-long poaching the cheese experiences before it is packed in salt and mint leaves.

Due to the saltiness of the cheese, the vinaigrette recipe does not call for salt. Also, the vinaigrette can be made ahead, but wait until you are ready to serve before adding the mint. Serves 4.

> 6 tablespoons olive oil, plus more for sautéing
>
> 2 tablespoons red wine vinegar
>
> 2 teaspoons French-style mustard, such as Dijon

1 garlic clove, minced

2 tablespoons fresh mint, chopped

Pepper to taste

8 slices halloumi cheese

4 cups seedless watermelon (about half of a small one), cut into bite-size chunks

1 medium Persian cucumber, cut into bite-size chunks

½ sweet onion, diced

Whisk together the oil, vinegar, mustard, garlic, and mint (if serving the dressing within the next few hours). Add pepper to taste.

Heat a nonstick pan over medium heat. Film with oil and add the halloumi slices. Brown on both sides. Remove from heat and keep warm.

Combine the watermelon, cucumber, and onion in a large bowl. Toss with the vinaigrette. Distribute the mixture to individual serving plates. Top with halloumi.

Barley Salad with Zucchini, Tomatoes, and Mint

The salt of the capers is an interesting foil to the fresh mint that is stirred in at the end of this recipe. Plus, this dish is the very definition of versatile: It is a comfort food when hot, a trusty potluck dish at room temperature, and a life saver when served cold the next day. No matter how you choose to eat this salad, stir in the mint right before you serve. Serves 4 as a main course or 8 as a side dish.

¼ cup pearled barley

½ teaspoon kosher salt, plus more to taste

1 cup water

2 tablespoons extra-virgin olive oil

1 medium onion, sliced

2 garlic cloves, minced

One 14-ounce can fire-roasted diced tomatoes

2 tablespoons brined capers, rinsed

3 medium zucchini, cubed

¼ cup fresh mint, chopped or shredded

Black pepper to taste

Place the barley, salt, and water in a saucepan. Bring to a boil, then simmer, stirring occasionally, until barley is tender and most of the liquid is absorbed, about 40 minutes. Drain any leftover water, and set barley aside to cool while you continue to cook the other parts of the recipe.

Heat the oil in a large skillet over medium heat. Add the onion and sauté until softened and turning a light golden color, about 10 minutes.

Clear a spot in the center of the skillet and drop in the garlic. Do not move it until it becomes fragrant, about 10 seconds. Then stir to combine with the onions. Add the tomatoes and capers. Bring to a boil.

Add the zucchini, then cover and reduce to a simmer. Stir occasionally until the zucchini is tender, about 15 minutes.

Remove lid and return the skillet to a boil. Stir occasionally while boiling off most of the liquid.

Stir in the barley, salt and pepper to taste, and mint if serving immediately. Otherwise, refrigerate the barley and zucchini mixture and stir in the mint when ready to serve.

Chicken with Lemon, Garlic, and Mint

This recipe is based on a version that the *San Francisco Chronicle* declared in 2006 to be one of the best recipes from the last ten years. Serves 4.

4 skinless, boneless chicken breasts

8–10 garlic cloves, chopped

1 cup lightly packed whole mint leaves, and more for garnish

2 lemons, juiced

2 tablespoons extra-virgin olive oil, and more for cooking

Salt and pepper to taste

½ cup white wine

1 cup chicken broth

1–2 tablespoons flour (optional)

1–2 teaspoons sugar (optional)

Place the chicken breasts, garlic, mint, lemon juice, 2 tablespoons olive oil, salt, and pepper in a resealable plastic bag to marinate overnight.

When ready to cook, remove the chicken from the marinade. Reserve the marinade. Remove the garlic and mint pieces stuck to the chicken, and return to the marinade. Dry the chicken to prevent spattering.

Heat a large pan over medium heat and film with olive oil. Sauté the chicken until cooked through, about 15 minutes. Monitor the heat to prevent scorching.

Remove the chicken and keep warm.

Pour off the fat from the pan, but do not wipe. Return to high heat and add the wine to deglaze it, scraping up the brown bits. After the wine has reduced by about half, add the chicken broth and marinade. Continue to reduce until the sauce is about 1 cup. You may add flour to thicken the sauce.

Taste the sauce and adjust the seasoning. If the lemons were especially tart, add some sugar.

Return the chicken, and any juices that collected, to the pan and heat through. Serve immediately, sprinkled with the extra mint.

Mint and Onion Bread

Dried mint withstands the heat in this recipe, infusing the bread with a sweetness that catches you by surprise. The sautéed onions are also sweet, but they firmly establish this bread as a savory baked good. Try it with havarti cheese or slices of boiled ham. Makes 1 loaf.

1 cup diced onion

4 tablespoons extra-virgin olive oil, divided

4 teaspoons active dry yeast

1 cup lukewarm water

1 teaspoon sugar

1 tablespoon kosher salt

3 ½–4 cups all-purpose flour

3 tablespoons dried mint

Topping:

1 tablespoon extra-virgin olive oil

Coarse sea salt and freshly ground black pepper to taste

Sauté the onions in a skillet over medium heat with ½ tablespoon oil. Cook until the pieces are translucent and beginning to brown. Remove from heat and set aside.

Mix yeast and warm water in a small bowl and stir in sugar. Let stand for at least 5 minutes. As the yeast activates, it should start to bubble up.

Combine salt, 2 tablespoons oil, and flour in the bowl of a standing electric mixer or food processor. Add the yeast mixture. With the mixer's motor on low speed or by pulsing the processor, mix until the dough just begins to come together.

Add the mint, onions, and any oil left in the skillet. Continue to process the dough until the mixture forms a smooth ball and is slightly sticky.

Place the dough in a bowl with ½ tablespoon oil, turn to coat, and cover with a tea towel. Let rise in a warm place until it doubles in volume, about 1 hour.

Punch down the dough, form it into a ball, and turn to re-coat it with oil. Cover and let dough rise again for about 45 minutes.

Punch it down again and place the dough on a baking pan oiled with another ½ tablespoon of oil. Use your hands to flatten and stretch the dough until it is about 6–8 inches wide. It does not have to reach the edges of the pan.

Brush the dough with the remaining oil and sprinkle with salt and pepper. Cover and let rise a final time for about 1 hour.

After the dough has risen about 40 minutes, preheat the oven to 400°F. Bake the bread for 25–30 minutes, until golden. The bread should sound hollow when the bottom is thumped. Let cool on a rack for at least 30 minutes before slicing.

Chocolate Mint Ricotta Cups

Most chocolate and mint desserts require adding a splash of crème de menthe. Here, the leaves are enough to flavor the cannoli-like filling. This is a perfect recipe to try with different kinds of mint. I would suggest ginger mint. Serves 5.

¾ cup whole milk ricotta cheese

3 ½ teaspoons granulated sugar

¼ teaspoon vanilla

1 lemon zested (about 1 teaspoon)

1 tablespoon packed, chopped mint leaves

1 teaspoon bittersweet chocolate, chopped fine

One 15-cup package miniature phyllo cup shells

Combine ricotta, sugar, vanilla, and lemon zest in a medium-size bowl. Mix thoroughly. Gently stir in the mint leaves.

Spoon a portion of the ricotta mixture into each phyllo cup. Then sprinkle with chocolate. Cover in plastic wrap and chill until ready to serve. They should be consumed the same day they are made.

Further Reading

Grieve, Mrs. M. *A Modern Herbal.* "Mints." Available online at http://botanical.com/botanical/mgmh/m/mints-39.html.

Hemphill, John, and Rosemary Hemphill. *What Herb Is That? How to Grow and Use the Culinary Herbs.* Mechanicsburg, PA: Stackpole Books, 1997.

Hollis, Sarah. *The Country Diary Herbal.* New York: Henry Holt & Co., 1990.

Kremezi, Aglaia. *The Foods of the Greek Islands: Cooking and Culture at the Crossroads of the Mediterranean.* New York: Houghton Mifflin, 2000.

McVicar, Jekka. *Jekka's Herb Cookbook.* Buffalo, NY: Firefly Books, 2011.

Potterton, David, ed. *Culpeper's Color Herbal.* New York: Sterling Publishing Co., 2007.

San Francisco Chronicle. "Top Recipe 1994: Sicilian Chicken with Lemon, Mint & Almonds." October 4, 2006. www .sfchronicle.com/recipes/article/Top-Recipe-1994-Sicilian -Chicken-with-Lemon-2468710.php.

Traunfeld, Jerry. *The Herbal Kitchen: Cooking with Fragrance and Flavor.* New York: HarperCollins, 2005.

Anne Sala *is a freelance journalist based in Minnesota. This summer, her two-year-old daughter declared the pot of mint on their deck to be her favorite herb. Every time she would pass it, she would tear off a leaf to eat or sniff. This constant attention resulted in the healthiest, happiest mint the Sala household has ever raised.*

Herbal Pestos and Spice Blends

❧ By Darcey Blue French ❧

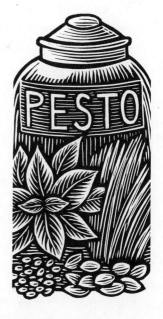

Culinary herbs are a popular and easy way to add flavor and interest to our daily meals, but did you realize that those same culinary herbs also pack a nutritional and health-boosting punch as well? Feeding ourselves is something we do three times a day, every single day of our lives, and our food should be our first medicine. Including health-boosting herbs in our daily fare is a flavorful and easy way to use herbal medicine as preventive medicine. It's easier to maintain health than regain it. I'm going to share with you several recipes that I use in my own herbal kitchen to add flavor and herbal healing benefits to my meals. They provide vitamins and minerals, improve digestion, strengthen immunity, and balance our well-being.

Herbal pestos are a delicious way to use fresh herbs that are abundant in your garden during spring and summer, and can be frozen for use later in the year. The spice blends use dried herbs and spices, which you can grow yourself and dry, or purchase in bulk. These blends can be placed on your table and used instead of table salt every day, all year long.

Herbal Health Pestos

These recipes use fresh herbs, which you can grow in your garden, wildcraft, or purchase in the fresh produce section of your grocery store. Dried herbs aren't a very good substitute for fresh herbs when it comes to pesto. If you can't find the herb in the recipe fresh, it's fine to substitute another herb you like. Almost all culinary herbs, as well as many weeds and medicinal herbs, can be used in pestos in varying quantities.

My favorites herbs include rosemary, sage, basil, oregano, monarda/beebalm, lemon verbena, peppermint/spearmint, nettles, dandelions, sweet clover, chives, marjoram, lovage, parsley, cilantro, fennel, hyssop, rose petals, and citrus/peel.

It's best to blend very strong-flavored herbs with other milder-tasting herbs when making pestos. For example, bitter dandelion leaves or sage can be combined with chives, parsley, or lemon verbena.

Also, pesto is very flexible, so you can use the ingredients you have on hand. Any nut or seed is fair game, depending on the flavor you want. Toasting the nuts ahead of time gives the pesto a fuller, more interesting taste. Try pumpkin seeds, almonds, walnuts, pecans, pine nuts, sunflower seeds, hazelnuts, or even cashews.

Cheeses are often added to pestos to boost flavor, and though I find these herbal pesto blends to be flavorful enough on their own, you can always try adding different hard or salted cheeses to your liking. Parmesan and Pecorino Romano are traditionally used in pestos, but you can try feta, asiago, or even goat cheese. Leave the cheese out if you are sensitive to dairy or want to support extra-healthy digestive function with your pestos. Serve your pestos over pasta, stirred in rice, or baked on fish, chicken, or potatoes. Or use as a topping for other foods or in homemade salad dressing.

Rosemary, Lemon, and Black Pepper Pesto

This piquant and perky pesto is perfectly delectable on potatoes, chicken, fish, pasta with white beans and summer squash, or stuffed into mushroom tops. Rosemary is a wonderful herbal ally for stimulating the digestion, clarifying the mind, and improving memory. Lemon and rosemary also both gently and effectively detoxify and stimulate healthy liver function.

½ cup toasted pepitas (pumpkin seeds)

2 cloves of garlic

2 cups fresh rosemary leaves, stripped off the stems

1 organic lemon, deseeded, chopped, with the peel

2 teaspoons black pepper, ground

½ teaspoon salt, or to taste

1 cup olive oil

Place pepitas, garlic, and rosemary in a blender or food processor and mince into a paste. Add chopped lemon, spices, and olive oil. Blend again. Serve immediately. Keeps in the fridge for 4–5 days, or freeze for long-term storage.

Fresh Stinging Nettle and Beebalm Pesto

Fresh nettles, available in the spring, grow wild in temperate climates or can be grown in your garden. Nettles are full of minerals like potassium, calcium, and iron, and pack a nutritious punch. Beebalm, or monarda *(M. punctata* or *M. didyma)*, are lovely garden flowers with brightly colored flowers that attract bees. Beebalm has a spicy and peppery taste much like oregano, but stronger! (Fresh oregano can be used instead if beebalm isn't available.)

This a wonderful spring tonic to nourish and stimulate the blood, the circulation, and the appetite. Beebalm has the added medicinal benefit of combating infections, so this is a great recipe to use if you have a cold or are recovering from a stomach bug.

3 cups fresh nettle leaves (remove from stems)

1 ½ cups pecans or walnuts

3 cloves garlic

½ cup Parmesan or Romano cheese (optional)

½ teaspoon salt, or to taste

1 cup beebalm leaves and flowers

1 ½–2 cups olive oil

Steam the nettle leaves for 30 to 60 seconds, then rinse immediately with cold water. Mince nuts, garlic, cheese, and salt in the processor until well chopped. Add nettles, beebalm, and olive oil. Pulse until well mixed. Serve over pasta, baked fish or chicken, or potatoes, or mix into sour cream or hummus for a delicious dip.

Dandelion and Chive Pesto

Dandelions are bitter and can be an acquired taste. This pesto mellows out the bitter flavor with snappy chives and lemon juice. Dandelion greens are full of potassium and support healthy liver and kidney function.

This is a perfect spring tonic to get your internal organs perked up, or for any time you want to give your organs a gentle cleanse and boost. Top fresh tomato and mozzarella slices with this dandelion pesto, or use it on baked fish, potatoes, or rice.

  2 cups fresh dandelion greens (wild or from the organic produce section)

  1 cup chopped chives or scallions

  1 ½ cups olive oil

  2 tablespoons lemon juice

  2 cloves of garlic

  1 cup toasted walnuts or pecans

  Salt and pepper to taste

Wash greens and chives, then pulse in the blender with all the ingredients until the mixture forms a smooth pesto consistency.

Lemon, Rose, and Mint Pesto

This delicate and fresh pesto reminds me of Middle Eastern feasts and markets. It has a totally unique flavor, which is best showcased with meals that don't have conflicting spicy or overwhelming flavors. This is one blend that can be adequately made with dried herbs if fresh aren't available. I recommend serving this pesto on baked fish or fragrant jasmine rice, or as a topping on hummus, yogurt, pita, cucumber salad, or lentils. This is a very cooling and mild blend of herbs that is perfect for hot summer evenings.

> 1 cup toasted piñon nuts (toasted almonds are also excellent)
>
> 1 tablespoon toasted sesame seeds
>
> 1 teaspoon cumin seed, toasted and ground
>
> 1 cup fresh rose petals
>
> 1 cup fresh mint leaves
>
> 1 cup olive oil
>
> Juice of 1 lemon
>
> ½ teaspoon salt

Toast nuts, sesame seeds, and cumin seeds. Set aside. Process and blend the nuts/seeds, then add remaining ingredients to the processor/blender. Blend until well incorporated. If you use dried herbs, please rehydrate in ¼ cup boiling stock or water before adding to the processor.

Digestion-Boosting Spice Blends

Spices are well known and used extensively in ethnic cooking. The flavors of India, Morocco, Thailand, China, and even Italy and France are captured by the spices and blends used in the preparation. In North America, our food tends to be bland or heavily focused on one flavor, usually salty or sweet. All the flavors are important for our digestive function, and we are especially missing the bitter and astringent flavors in our food. Spices make our food interesting and enjoyable, and they improve our ability to digest our food properly. When used regularly, spices can ease indigestion, heartburn, or gas. I like to say, "Spice is the variety of life." If you are not familiar with using varied spices in your cooking, these blends are a perfect place to start, and can be added to food at the table, just like salt or pepper.

These spice blends are meant to be used frequently, even daily, and can be stored for longer periods of time, and made in larger batches to keep on hand. All spice blends are made with culinary herbs, often garlic, black pepper, salt, chives, lemon peels, cumin, chiles, etc. But these recipes have an added boost of medicinal herbs that can stimulate and improve digestion, immune health, energy, and nutrition when used daily in your meals.

It is quite easy to make your own spice blends, using herbs you like. But start off with small batches when creating new blends, so you don't end up with a large quantity of a blend you don't like. Try to incorporate spices/herbs that have all of the six flavors (pungent/spicy, bitter, sour, astringent, salty, and sweet). Use a light hand with the spicy, bitter, and salty flavors in your blends, as they can overpower the flavor in large quantities.

I prefer to buy my spices and seeds as whole as possible, and powder them myself in a spice grinder. This preserves the flavor and medicinal benefits much longer than the pre-ground spices, which have been sitting on a shelf or in a cabinet for unknown lengths of time. Try ethnic markets to buy whole spices if you can't find them at the supermarket, or you can buy them online from herb suppliers like Mountain Rose Herbs or Frontier Herbs.

Za'atar

This is a traditional spice blend from the Middle East that features sumac berries, which is a commonly found weedy shrub/tree in many parts of the United States. You can harvest your own sumac berries in late summer or early fall, or purchase them at Middle Eastern or ethnic markets. I've modified the traditional recipe to reflect balance and health in digestion. This spice blend is delicious over hummus, steamed vegetables, rice, salads, or baked fish or chicken.

½ cup sesame seeds, toasted

½ cup oregano leaves, dry

¼ cup nettle leaf, dry

¼ cup rose petals, dry

¼ cup peppermint leaf, dry

1 tablespoon fennel seed

½ cup sumac powder

1 tablespoon aleppo chile (or red chile flakes)

2 teaspoons sea salt

Toast the sesame seeds in a dry skillet and cool. Mix all the dry herbs and grind briefly in a spice grinder. Don't powder them completely, just break them up and incorporate them evenly. Grind salt and toasted sesame seeds together. Blend all ingredients and store in an airtight shaker or jar.

Earth and Sea Zingy Blend

This spice blend is a nourishing topping for all kinds of foods, and boosts the mineral and vitamin content of whatever you sprinkle it on. It uses herbal ingredients from both land and sea. The herbs included also are considered adaptogens and help the body handle stress better, boost immune health, and improve energy.

   ½ cup toasted nori flakes

   1 tablespoon dulse flakes

   ½ cup nettle leaf

   1 tablespoon black pepper, ground

   1 tablespoon schizandra berry, ground

   2 tablespoons dried shiitake mushroom, ground

Grind all ingredients finely in a spice grinder. Mix together and shake abundantly for a burst of flavor, mineral nutrition, and an energy boost.

Six-Flavor Churna

In Ayurveda, the traditional healing system of India, it is said that there are six flavors: bitter, sour, salty, pungent, astringent, and sweet. We need all six flavors in every meal and every day to be fully satisfied and nourished and to digest our food properly. Churnas are often made with herbs and spices to improve digestion, and add the flavors missing from prepared foods. This is my version, which contains all six flavors in a tasty balance. Sprinkle this on all your meals in small quantities to improve digestion.

   1 teaspoon sea salt

   1 teaspoon rose petal powder

   1 teaspoon ginger root powder

   ½ teaspoon licorice root powder

   1 teaspoon rosehip powder

   ½ teaspoon dandelion root powder

Mix all ingredients together and store in an airtight shaker or jar. You can powder your own herbs in a spice grinder if you do not have powdered herbs on hand.

Darcey Blue French *is a shamanic and clinical herbalist and wildcrafter of plant medicines. She calls herself a devotee of all that is sacred on this wild, beautiful earth. She learns from the plants and listens for the quiet, intuitive knowing of a plant communicating to her its love, its medicine, its nature enveloped and rooted in the magic of the natural world—the place where the heart hears what is being said. She is here to dive deep into the wild world and to experience, to sense, to taste, to feel the magic of the plants and the wisdom of spirit within each of us. Darcey lives and works in the southwestern deserts and mountains of Tucson, Arizona, where she maintains her private healing practice and offers an Herbal Medicine CSA, a shamanic herbal apprenticeship, medicinal plant walks, and plant medicine retreats. She was trained in clinical herbalism/ nutrition at the North American Institute for Medical Herbalism. Visit Darcey online at www.shamanaflora.com.*

A Sprig of Parsley

⤞ By Elizabeth Barrette ⤝

Parsley (*Petroselinum crispum*) is a plant of Mediterranean origin. It measures about a foot in height and spread. Gardeners grow it as an herb, a spice, and a vegetable. Technically a biennial, it forms a rosette of tripinnate leaves and a taproot that stores food over the winter. Then it flowers and sets seed in the second year. The flowers appear in umbels of tiny white to yellow blossoms. However, many people treat this herb as an annual in cooler climates.

There are two main types of leaf parsley, divided by leaf shape. Curly leaf parsley (*P. crispum* var. *crispum*) has deeply crinkled leaves. This type has a sharper flavor and is most often used as a garnish. Italian parsley (*P. crispum* var. *neapolitanum*) has flat

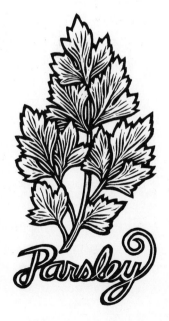

leaves similar to the wild species. This variety is easier to cultivate and more tolerant of variations in rain and sun. It has a mellower but rich flavor that blends well in recipes, and is more fragrant and less bitter than curly parsley.

Then there is root parsley. Hamburg parsley (*P. crispum* var. *tuberosum*) produces a thick, edible taproot. This vegetable is popular in Central and Eastern European recipes, where it is used similar to carrots. It may be added to stews and casseroles or eaten raw as a snack food.

Cultivation

Parsley grows best in moist, well-worked soil. Plant as soon as the garden can be worked, as this herb does better in the cool weather of spring and fall. It prefers partial shade. During summer, extra sun protection may help the plants stay healthy.

Garden stores typically sell parsley as plants, often in packs of four to six. This herb transplants well, so plants are a good choice for small amounts. It's also convenient if you want several different types of parsley. Young plants transplant pretty well. Mature parsley dislikes being moved and may sulk for weeks before putting out new leaves. Try transplanting on a wet day, and take as large a root ball as feasible.

Seed may be sown in prepared soil by drills or broadcasting. Take care not to bury the seeds too deep, no more than a quarter inch. Drill holes should be placed a foot apart. If you want to grow a lot of parsley, use seed. A succession of sowings will be necessary for a sustained harvest, spaced two months apart, such as February, April, and June.

Once the seedlings sprout, weed carefully. Thin plants eight to twelve inches apart. Parsley needs space and dislikes crowding. Water generously in hot weather. A layer of mulch around the plants, but not touching them, helps to retain moisture and keep the soil cooler.

After plants reach at least six inches high, harvest by picking individual sprigs as needed. If the leaves become coarse in summer, cut off the whole top about two inches above the soil, then water heavily around the base. Tender new leaves will sprout from the roots.

Curly parsley may be overwintered with protection. It is so hardy that it often survives into December even when exposed. Protect the plants with a hoop tunnel, cold frame, or unheated greenhouse. You don't need anything fancy. You can stretch plastic sheeting over improvised support such as stacked tires or hay bales, or use old windows propped up with bricks.

Cooking

Parsley is an excellent source of vitamin K, vitamin C, and vitamin A. It's a good source of folic acid and iron. It has very few calories. The flavonoids in parsley perform as antioxidants, protecting human cells from damage.

In Central and Eastern Europe, curly leaf parsley is chopped and sprinkled atop various recipes. It is most popular on potatoes, rice, and vegetable stews. Some people also add chopped parsley to fish, chicken, goose, lamb chops, or beef steaks. It can be used in sandwiches or salads.

In Southern and Central Europe, cooks often use a *bouquet garni* consisting of bundled herbs that may be either fresh (tied with string) or dried (in a muslin bag or tea ball). This provides flavor to various soups, sauces, and stocks. Parsley customarily appears in the fresh version; it can be dried but has much less flavor then. A popular combination is sweet basil, parsley, sage, tarragon, rosemary, and thyme.

Parsley contributes to several distinctive sauces and condiments. French cuisine features *persillade*, a mixture of garlic and parsley chopped together. Italian cuisine offers two more. *Gremolata* is a blend of parsley, garlic, and lemon zest served with veal stew. *Salsa verde* combines parsley, capers, anchovies, garlic, and vinegar-soaked bread. It accompanies such dishes as *bollito misto* or fish. *Chimichurri* is a South American condiment similar to pesto but based on parsley instead of basil, with garlic, oil, and vinegar. It is customarily served with steak.

Dried parsley doesn't retain its flavor as well as other herbs do, but it still has its uses. Throw a tablespoon or so into a pot of soup or stew and it reconstitutes pretty well. It also works nicely in mashed potatoes or stuffing. You can add parsley flakes to most combinations of dried herbs if you're making a rub or sprinkle blend. Dried parsley also has the advantage of lasting much longer than fresh.

Parsley Recipes

Caramelized Root Vegetables

4 carrots

2 parsley roots

2 parsnips

2 Yukon Gold potatoes

1 cup pearl onions

Water

2 tablespoons buckwheat or sage honey

1 tablespoon parsley flakes

Sea salt

Ground white pepper

Preheat oven to 350°F. Scrub the carrots, parsley roots, parsnips, and potatoes. Cut the ends off. Chop the vegetables into bite-size chunks. Add them, along with the pearl onions, to a large baking dish.

Put just enough water into the baking dish to cover the bottom. Drizzle 2 tablespoons buckwheat or sage honey over the vegetables. (These are dark honeys with a nutty, herbal flavor.) Sprinkle with parsley flakes. Add sea salt and ground white pepper to taste.

Cook for half an hour to an hour, stirring occasionally, until all the vegetables are tender when poked with a fork. If they start sticking to the bottom, add a little more water.

Terrific Tabbouleh

   1 cup bulgur (cracked wheat)

   2 cups boiling water

   1 cup cherry tomatoes

   2 cucumbers

   3 green onions

   3 cloves garlic

   1 bunch fresh parsley (about 1 cup chopped)

   ⅓ cup fresh mint leaves

   2 lemons (about ¼ cup juice)

   1 teaspoon sea salt

   ½ teaspoon multicolored peppercorns

   ½ cup extra-virgin olive oil

In a large bowl, place the bulgur and cover it with 2 cups boiling water. Soak for half an hour.

Rinse and quarter the cherry tomatoes. Peel and chop the cucumbers. Chop the green onions, both the white and the green parts, discarding the very end with the fuzzy roots. Peel and mince the garlic cloves. Chop the parsley and the mint. Combine all these vegetables in a mixing bowl.

Juice the lemons and add the juice to the mixing bowl.

With a mortar and pestle, grind together the sea salt and multicolored peppercorns. Add that to the mixing bowl.

Drain the bulgur and squeeze out any excess water. Add the bulgur to the mixing bowl. Pour in the olive oil. Toss thoroughly to combine. Refrigerate for at least 4 hours.

Toss tabbouleh again after refrigeration. Transfer to a serving bowl.

Sunny Parsley Butter

8 tablespoons (1 stick) unsalted butter

Zest of 1 lemon

2 tablespoons lemon juice

¼ teaspoon sea salt

¼ cup finely chopped fresh parsley

Set butter on counter to warm to room temperature.

Zest and juice the lemon. Save the zest and 2 tablespoons of juice in a small bowl. Mix in the sea salt.

Place the butter in a mixing bowl. Beat with an electric mixer or by hand until light and fluffy. In small amounts, add the lemon juice, zest, and salt mixture. Beat in the parsley, allowing time to combine before adding more. Allow to sit for half an hour to an hour so the flavors can blend; the longer you let it stay at room temperature, the stronger the flavors get.

Scoop the parsley butter onto a sheet of waxed paper. Gently roll and press until it forms a small log. Twist the ends closed to seal. Chill until firm, preferably overnight. This will keep for about 2 weeks in the refrigerator.

Parsley butter makes an excellent bread spread. Use it for topping fish, chicken, or cooked vegetables. It is especially good over asparagus or corn on the cob.

Winter Pesto

1 bunch flat leaf parsley

4 garlic cloves

¼ teaspoon sea salt

½ teaspoon green peppercorns

1 cup black walnuts

½ cup grated pecorino cheese

½ cup extra-virgin olive oil

Coarsely chop the parsley and garlic cloves. With a mortar and pestle, grind together the sea salt and green peppercorns.

Into a food processor, put the parsley, garlic, sea salt, green pepper, walnuts, and pecorino cheese. Pulse to combine. Add the olive oil in small amounts. Scrape down the sides of the bowl as necessary, then pulse again, until the ingredients are combined. If you don't have a food processor, you can make this pesto with a mortar and pestle—it just takes more effort to grind everything to paste.

Winter pesto may be served immediately or stored in the refrigerator for a few days in a sealed bowl. It makes an excellent condiment for toast, sandwiches, or pasta.

Visionary Juice

1 ½ pounds carrots

1 bunch parsley

2 apples

1 tablespoon local honey

Cut the ends off the carrots, scrub them clean, and cut into chunks. Coarsely chop the parsley. Core the apples and slice them. Run them all through a juicer or other appliance until liquefied. (With a food processor or blender, you'll probably need to strain the results.)

Stir in 1 tablespoon local honey. Enjoy! The vitamins in carrots and parsley are excellent for supporting healthy eyesight, and the apples improve the flavor.

Other Uses

In the garden, parsley makes a beautiful border plant with a relatively compact form. The deep green of curly parsley tends to look nicer. Flat leaf parsley has a paler color and a more airy appearance. Either can work in a pot of mixed herbs for a container garden.

Note that parsley is the favored food of the parsley worm caterpillar, which matures into the beautiful black swallowtail butterfly (*Papilio polyxenes*). The caterpillars are striped in black, white, yellow, and green; they have orange "horns" that emerge when startled. If you are concerned about caterpillars eating your garden, consider planting some parsley especially for them in a place where you won't mind having the leaves nibbled. It's easy to move the baby butterflies from your kitchen herb garden to your butterfly garden. Butterflies are beneficial insects that pollinate flowers and make the outdoors more enjoyable. They also represent the element of air, for those of you into elemental gardening.

Medicinally, parsley helps with feminine complaints. It stimulates menstruation, relieves cramps and bloating, and provides iron to make up for the lost blood. Fresh parsley tea is one good medicinal application. Another use for parsley is soothing digestion; it blends well with other digestive herbs, such as sage, oregano, and rosemary. Either fresh or dried parsley will work for this. Green parsley may be chewed to freshen the breath, which is worth remembering after a nice dinner out when you have no toothbrush but there's a sprig of garnish left on your plate.

In ancient Greece, parsley was associated with success but also with the Underworld. Winners were sometimes crowned with parsley instead of laurel. The herb was sacred to Persephone and to Charon. It was used in funeral rites and bouquets.

In the language of flowers, parsley can signify useful knowledge, entertainment, festivity, a banquet, or lasting pleasure. It appears on dining invitations and in tabletop bouquets.

Elizabeth Barrette *has been involved with the Pagan community for more than twenty-four years. She served as Managing Editor of* PanGaia *for eight years and Dean of Studies at the Grey School of Wizardry for four years. She has written columns on beginning and intermediate Pagan practice, Pagan culture, and Pagan leadership. Her book* Composing Magic: How to Create Magical Spells, Rituals, Blessings, Chants, and Prayers *explains how to combine writing and spirituality. She lives in central Illinois, where she has done much networking with Pagans in her area, such as coffeehouse meetings and* open sabbats. *Her other public activities feature Pagan picnics and science fiction conventions. She enjoys magical crafts, historic religions, and gardening for wildlife. Her other writing fields include speculative fiction, gender studies, and social and environmental issues. Visit her blog* The Wordsmith's Forge, *http://ysabetwordsmith.livejournal .com, or her website* PenUltimate Productions, *http://penultimate productions.weebly.com. Her coven site with extensive Pagan materials is* Greenhaven Tradition, http://greenhaventradition.weebly.com.

Herbal Pantry Staples: Time Savers with Great Flavors

⇒ By Doreen Shababy ⇐

Keeping these herb-inspired, fruit-infused, flavor-loaded pantry staples will surround you with the aura of a seasoned Kitchen Goddess. You will turn plain biscuits and cold chicken into remarkable fare, raise eyebrows over the humble mac and cheese, and create a stampede from a simple pot of beans. Oh, we're gonna have fun!

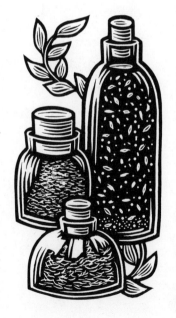

You can make most of these easy and family-friendly pantry staples at home. Do you grow your own herbs? Frequent the farmers' market? If not, you can still buy quality dried herbs through many reliable sources, and many fruits and berries can be found locally. Other items, such as vinegar or butter, are the foundation for some of these creations and are readily available. My kitchen is organic. I highly recommend you move in that direction, too.

Herb and Spice Blends

How many times have you picked up that dusty bottle of Italian herb blend and put it right back on the shelf because the contents looked and smelled (and no doubt tasted) equally dusty? Well, no more, my dears. You will make your own blend based on my recipe, and you will tweak it to your own taste if you wish.

Preparing these herbal seasoning blends is easy. Simply put all the ingredients for a given recipe in a large mixing bowl, gently crush together with your fingers to blend, and spoon into little spice bottles—you will even have a couple extra for gifting. All ingredients called for are dried, chopped/crushed herbs unless otherwise noted. Also, my suggestions are only suggestions. Feel free to experiment, and enjoy the process.

Italian Seasoning Blend

  ½ cup each basil, oregano, and parsley

  1 tablespoon each sage leaf, fennel seed (whole), and crushed red pepper flakes

  1 teaspoon garlic granules

Sprinkle over "pizza-tillas"! Makes about 2 cups.

French Mediterranean Blend

  4 tablespoons fennel seeds, bruised (do not completely crush)

  3 tablespoons thyme leaf

2 tablespoons each rosemary, sweet marjoram, and summer savory

1 tablespoon each lavender buds, sage leaf, and sweet basil

1 teaspoon powdered bay leaf, if available (if not, just toss a bay leaf into the dish)

Roasted potatoes are just the beginning for this fragrant blend. Makes about 1 cup.

English Mixed Herbs

4 tablespoons each chives, parsley, tarragon, and thyme

Use this blend with roast lamb or pork or stuffed mushrooms. This recipe courtesy of Mrs. M. Grieve. Makes about 1 cup.

Cajun Spice Blend

½ cup thyme

¼ cup each garlic granules, onion flakes, oregano, paprika, and sea salt

1 tablespoon each cayenne and black pepper

I love this on popcorn. Makes about 2 cups.

Sesame Nettle Sprinkle

1 cup toasted white sesame seeds, cooled, then coarsely ground

¼ cup dried crushed nettle leaf

1 teaspoon sea salt

Steamed veggies and cooked grains become nutty with this blend, which is similar to Japanese gomasio. Makes about 1 cup.

Just in time for slow-cooker season, the next two herbal blends are for spicing up hearty bean soups. The first one features kelp leaf (found at natural food stores), which naturally tenderizes the beans, and the second blend is a wild and crazy mix of herbs and aromatic seeds. Use 1–2 tablespoons blend to a pot o' beans, or to your taste.

Greens for Beans

½ cup chopped, crushed, or snipped kelp (also known as kombu, konbu, or nori; don't use powdered—ew!)

½ cup dried, crushed nettle leaf

2 tablespoons each sweet marjoram, oregano, sage leaf, and summer savory

1 teaspoon dried ginger root powder

Makes about 1 ½ cups.

Herb Mix for Bean Soup

1 cup dried crushed parsley

¾ cup summer savory

½ cup cumin seed

¼ cup each fennel seed, caraway seed, dill seed, coriander seed, and sweet basil leaf

2 tablespoons each celery seed, thyme leaf, sage leaf, oregano, rosemary, lavender, and sweet marjoram

1 tablespoon cayenne pepper

Makes about 2 ½ cups.

Flavored Vinegars

Flavored vinegar is another useful pantry staple, whether for salad dressing or to jazz up the potlikker from a slow-cooked venison roast. The ubiquitous raspberry vinegar is seen everywhere for good reason—the taste is divine! You can even add a splash of it to ice water for an old-fashioned Raspberry Shrub. Some other ideas for flavored vinegars include spicy peach, blueberry, or lime with cilantro and mint. Following are the basic instructions.

Fruit-Flavored Vinegar

Fill a freshly washed Mason jar halfway with chunks of fresh or frozen fruit (leave berries whole, except strawberries), then cover to fill with the 5% acidity vinegar of your choice—plain, cider, or wine vinegar. Add a sprig of this or a stem of that for extra flavor, if desired. Cover with wax paper and a clean lid, label, and date. Swirl gently every day for 2–4 weeks depending on desired strength (it's okay to taste along the way). Then carefully strain into a cleanly washed bottle, and cover with a cap. Label and date, and use within a year.

Herb-Flavored Vinegar

Making herb-flavored vinegar is pretty much the same process as with fruit, and you can add small amounts of citrus juice or sweetener to either type if you wish. Just be sure that all your equipment is super clean. In my book *The Wild & Weedy Apothecary*, I offer details on three different methods for making herbal vinegars, each with their own practicalities.

I sometimes use flavored vinegar in place of wine in cooking. Of course the volume is much less, but the flavor is concentrated, and you may need to add more liquid to the dish to make up the difference. Just add several glugs of vinegar to whatever you are simmering; I usually add some to my chicken soup stock. And don't forget the mother of all vinegars, the intriguingly sweet balsamic vinegar of Modena, Italy—accept no substitutes. I use it all the time.

Pickles and Relishes

Jar food is making a beautiful comeback, although among home canners it never took a break. These pantry staples turn a sleepy Saturday afternoon and a plate of cold meat into a smorgasbord when served with cheese and crackers, apples, pears, or a fresh veggie plate. You can also turn steamed veggies into easy refrigerator pickles. Place veggies in a clean jar, and fill to cover with one of the flavored vinegars you made for just such an occasion. Add a glug of olive oil, a pinch of salt, and maybe sugar, then cover and refrigerate for three days. Eat within a week, if they last that long.

Don't overlook grocery store shelves either; a jar of marinated artichokes can transform many ordinary foods. How about baked macaroni and cheese Mediterranean-style? Use part mozzarella with other cheeses, then add the drained, chopped artichokes, some roasted red peppers, and a few capers. As my Grandma Rose would have said, "This is too good for kids!"

While I can't give you all the details on preserving (canning) pickled veggies in this article, approved methods for preserving are available through the University of Georgia Cooperative

Extension website, http://nchfp.uga.edu, which is my personal go-to for preserving questions.

Jams and Jellies

These foods add sweet, intense flavor and are useful for more than PB&Js. For instance, apricot jam makes a fabulous base for barbeque sauce. Even jellied cranberry sauce can be melted down and doctored into a type of catsup. Don't be afraid to experiment with flavors—the fruity sweet accepts the spicy heat with delicious results, and you'll use less sugar making a BBQ sauce if you start with jam.

Seasoned Bread Crumbs

Make your own bread crumbs in the blender or food processor. My Gramma Lil used to make hers with a hand grinder— I loved helping! Keep them in the freezer, and remember to label and date. Mix plain crumbs with Italian seasoning blend, chopped nuts, or grated cheese, and use on gratins such as that grown-up mac and cheese, for breading, or wherever else you use breadcrumbs. In my experience, starting with a hearty loaf of Italian bread and drying it in thin slices makes the best crumbs. Now that my kitchen is wheat-free, this is a bit of a challenge, but a grainy gluten-free loaf is acceptable in place of the white bread (I didn't say it was the same, though). I have learned to use nuts in place of bread crumbs for some gluten-free recipes, and they also stand in for cheese, too, since one of us in the household is allergic to dairy. It's an interesting journey.

Flavored Butters

These babies take home the blue ribbon as undisputed Queen of the Rodeo, as flavored butter is a sure way to spread the love on just about anything that isn't still moving. Whether you add herbs, nuts, cheese, dried fruits, fresh citrus peel, kala-yum-mata olives, or aromatic roots, flavored butters are a splendid way to accent the simple beauty of steamed vegetables. "Softened" butter means butter that has been at room temperature for a few hours, not melted butter. Most of these recipes (except the first one) are easily prepared by mixing all the ingredients in a large bowl with a wooden spoon.

Raspberry Butter

> 1 cup (2 sticks) butter, softened
>
> ½ cup raspberry purée (from unsweetened frozen berries, sieved for seeds)
>
> 1–2 tablespoons honey

Put all ingredients into the blender and mix well, scraping sides often to blend. Spoon into a pretty crock, or make a log using wax paper to roll. Chill before serving with biscuits, scones, or just your spoon. Makes about 1½ cups.

Garlicky Dill Butter

> 1 cup (2 sticks) butter, softened
>
> ¼ cup chopped fresh dill leaf
>
> 3–4 cloves chopped garlic

This is one of my favorites and is good on veggies, potatoes, and fish. You could also add a squeeze of lemon juice if you wish. Makes about 1 cup.

Citrus Butter with Basil and Tarragon

    1 cup (2 sticks) butter, softened

    Juice of ¼ each lemon, lime, and orange

    1 tablespoon each minced basil and tarragon leaf

    ½ teaspoon salt

    ½ teaspoon sugar (optional)

    Pinch fresh ground pepper

This butter is very good with asparagus, fish, and chicken. Makes about 1 cup.

During the Middle Ages, butter was wrapped in sorrel leaves, placed into crocks, then covered with salted water for keeping. In modern kitchens, small serving crocks or decorated logs make a nice presentation, and the butter will keep for about ten days in the refrigerator. You can also pack these "compound" butters into small freezer containers and freeze to keep for several weeks, which is very convenient. Ways to use flavored butter include spreading them on breads, over hot breakfast cereal or rice, over pasta or soups, and, of course, with steamed veggies. Just in case you need an idea for using the butter, try this next recipe.

Puff Pastry Twists

Thaw 1 package frozen puff pastry for 20 minutes. Preheat oven according to package directions (medium hot). Cut dough into finger-width strips across the short way. Brush with flavored butter, then twist dough like a ribbon and place on a lined baking sheet. Bake for 8–10 minutes or until golden. Let cool slightly before serving.

Let's Get Together Again Soon

I wish there was space to share more recipes! Find your own favorites and keep them handy for making flavorful family meals easier to prepare.

Sources Consulted

A Kitchen Witch's Cookbook by Patricia Telesco

A Modern Herbal by Mrs. M. Grieve

The Cooking of Southwest France by Paula Wolfert

Dairy Hollow House Soup & Bread Cookbook by Crescent Dragonwagon

Flavored Butters by Offerico Maoz

Healing Wise by Susun Weed

The Herbal Palate Cookbook by Maggie Oster and Sal Gilbertie

The Herbal Pantry by Emelie Tolley and Chris Mead

Recipe Goldmine, www.recipegoldmine.com/spread/raspberry-butter.html.

The Wild & Weedy Apothecary by Doreen Shababy

Doreen Shababy *is the author of* The Wild & Weedy Apothecary. *She has been using, growing, and teaching others about herbs for decades, and she is also involved with energy work. Please visit her blog at www.thewildnweedykitchen.blogspot.com.*

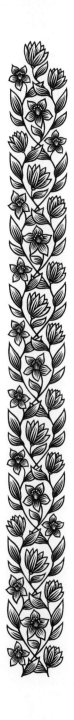

Herbs for
Health and
Beauty

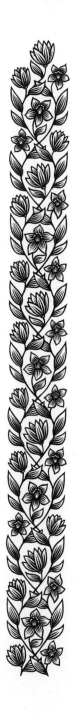

Back to Balance: Making Herbal Tonics

❧ By Dallas Jennifer Cobb ❧

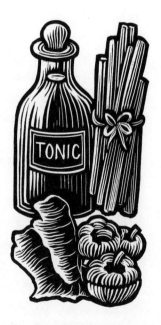

L iving in a fast-paced world, we're bombarded daily with myriad stressors. Whether it's loud noise, air pollution, a failing stock market, or international conflicts, we can be thrown out of balance internally by external happenings. Add to these the everyday stresses of managing our personal lives, time, money, families, and relationships, and it's no wonder we are dying from stress-related ailments. We are out of balance.

While we think that experiences are things that happen around us or outside of us, biologists have found that it is our internal responses that constitute the majority of our "lived experience." In response to the perceived outside experience, chemical messages are produced and dumped into the bloodstream and surrounding tissues by the endocrine system, which includes the pituitary gland, thyroid gland, parathyroid gland, adrenal glands, pancreas, ovaries, and testes, and to a lesser degree the gut, our fatty tissues, and the kidneys. It's their response that creates our internalized "experience."

Working with the nervous system and immune system, the endocrine response attempts to help the body cope with perceived external stressors by sending messages to specific parts of the body to stimulate preparedness.

In many situations, the endocrine response is needed and helpful. The chemical messages stimulate cellular growth and repair, the process of digestion, homeostasis (that delicate internal state of balance), and sexual attraction, arousal, and reproduction.

But with so much going on around us, and so many external stressors, imagine how many chemical messages are stimulated within us every day, and how easily our systems can be thrown out of balance, and how in this state diseases can manifest and grow.

Like nature, the human body always strives to return to homeostasis. Homeostasis is defined as "constant stability," coming from the Greek words *homeo* and *stasis*. Homeostasis, in part, is maintained by the liver, kidneys, hypothalamus, the endocrine system, and the autonomic nervous system, which all work together to regulate energy, temperature, blood pH levels, water levels, essential salt and mineral balances, and how the body metabolizes carbohydrates (fuel) and toxins. The process of returning to homeostasis is the set of complex interactions that enable the body to respond to and compensate for external and internal changes.

Tonics

A tonic is a nourishing formula that tones, builds, and strengthens, facilitating a return to homeostasis. Some of the herbs used in tonics act subtly on the endocrine organs, aiding them in the process of returning to and maintaining homeostasis (facilitating digestion by regulating the production of enzymes, for example). Other herbs act directly on internalized stressors that lay within the body (like ridding the digestive tract of worms).

While I learned the basics of making tonics in Jamaica, using Jamaican herbs, I have continued the practice since returning to my home in Canada. Jamaica herbs are widely available worldwide, and many are popular, easily accessible spices like ginger, cinnamon, and pimento. This article includes information on the Jamaican herbs, and herbs and spices that are widely available in North America. These can be used to make herbal tonics that will help to bring us "back to balance," aiding the body in its instinctual drive to return to homeostasis.

As there are many external and internal stressors, there are also many different tonics that can help bring us back to balance. The following are a variety of recipes for tonics specific to different stressors. But don't feel limited by these. As you learn about your particular kinds of stress, take time to identify the ingredients that will facilitate homeostasis. With the help of a skilled herbalist, you can create an herbal tonic specifically prescribed for you. Consider this article as a starting place as you begin to gather the information you need to get back to balance.

Jamaican Traditions

Living for almost five years in Jamaica, I learned a lot about Jamaican herbal tonics. Most people made them, preserved them, and even buried them in their yard for careful curing over time. These tonics were herbal remedies designed to help the body overcome the effects of stress, illness, exhaustion, and overwork and to restore internal balance. Some tonics were stimulants, and others were relaxants, prescribed for very specific stressors. Each tonic contained different herbs, and had its own unique signature and effect. Rooted in the traditional knowledge of herbs and roots common to their homelands, Jamaicans widely used these tonics in the prevention and treatment of ailments.

Many of the Jamaican herbs used to make tonics have wonderful names. Chaney root (*Smilax balbisiana*) is commonly used in energy tonics. Known as an antidote for anemia and fatigue, it increases red blood cell production and neutralizes blood pH levels. It is also used in pain-relief remedies and in aphrodisiac tonics.

Sarsaparilla root (*Smilax regelii*) is used for pain relief, to get rid of worms, and to support the strong functioning of the liver and colon in elimination and purification. Known for balancing hormones, it is a regular addition to aphrodisiac and anti-aging tonics.

Ginger root (*Zingiber officinale*) is widely used to promote strong digestion, emulating the digestive enzymes naturally found in the gut. It is also widely used to relieve nausea and morning sickness. Known for its antiviral qualities, ginger root helps to kill viruses and is used to treat flu. A tasty inclusion to any tonic, it adds a bit of zing taste-wise and a spicy bite.

Ginger is frequently used in combination with other bitter-tasting herbs.

Pimento (*Pimenta dioica*), also known as allspice, is not just a good-tasting spice but is an herb renowned for its warming and soothing qualities. It has been used to reduce inflammation and to encourage the production of good flora within the body. It is commonly included in energy tonics and vitality boosters.

Cinnamon (*Cinnamomum verum*) is used in Long Life Tonic and a wide variety of anti-aging compounds. It is said to help lower blood sugar and cholesterol levels and to increase alertness and circulation. Cinnamon is widely used in the treatment of sugar diabetes in Jamaica.

The tonics made from these herbs and many others have equally colorful names that often bear clues to their prescribed action: Long Life, Higher Level, Chill, Front End Loader, and Tear Down de Fence, to name a few.

Expelling Parasites

We don't often think about parasites here in North America, but in Jamaica I learned the value of periodically consuming tonics to expel parasites. These include invasive bacteria, life forms, and worms that can thrive within a human system.

With so much fruit growing in Jamaica, it was common to gorge on mangoes throughout their season. At the end of mango season, people commonly consumed a vermifuge, or anthelmintic (a substance that kills intestinal worms and helps to expel them), ridding the body of any worms that may have been acquired through mango consumption.

In North America, we commonly worm our pet cats and dogs, but do we ever consider our own needs for addressing internal parasites? Worms can enter the human digestive system through the mouth, lay eggs in the stomach and intestines, and eventually spread to affect other organs. Worms that commonly affect humans include roundworms, pinworms, whipworms, tapeworms, and hookworms.

The most commonly used Jamaican tonic with vermifuge qualities is a combination of the juice of two limes puréed with the gel from a large aloe vera leaf (*Aloe barbadensis*). This concoction was prepared fresh and consumed morning and night on an empty stomach, for three days, facilitating the expulsion of worms and their eggs/larvae.

Additionally, there are many simple, widely available food sources that work. These include pumpkin seeds (*Cucurbita pepo*), pineapple (*Ananas comosus*) and papaya (*Carica papaya*). Common herbs best known for getting rid of parasites are black walnut husk (*Juglans nigra*), wormwood (*Artemisia absinthium*), and cloves (*Syzygium aromaticum*).

Energy Tonics

The body experiences both acute and chronic stress. Acute stress is situational. For example, in a crisis situation, the sympathetic nervous system prepares the body to be ready for "fight or flight" through a complex variety of chemical messages. The adrenal glands produce cortisol and adrenaline and a variety of other chemical messages. These are dumped into the bloodstream and stimulate an increase in glucose levels, an increased heart rate, dilated air passages, and constricted blood vessels. Their positive effect is that we can jump up and quickly respond to the perceived threat. Their often negative side effects include hyperventilation and dizziness.

After the stressful situation has passed, we often feel a huge let-down feeling as our system runs out of the chemical messages that we were running on. We can feel situational exhaustion, which in extreme cases can cause a shock response, where people's bodies literally shut down.

Chronic stress tends to be something that stretches out over time, and is more lifestyle-based. When we don't sleep enough, sleep poorly, or eat foods that don't fuel the body effectively, we can get run down. With our modern addictions to caffeine and stimulants, we often have low-level chronic overproduction of stress by-products. For example, coffee consumption stimulates the production of cortisol. After long periods of cortisol-production stimulation, the body can become exhausted. This is chronic stress.

Whether acutely or chronically, stress can have a negative effect on our body, and the feeling of exhaustion is a common response. One of the first remedies for exhaustion is the elimination of stress-producing situations and substances, where possible. But we cannot always control these. Sure, we can quit drinking coffee and switch to herbal tea, and this will help, but most of us can't just quit our jobs regardless of the stress level.

Combating Stress

In Jamaica, marijuana (*Cannabis sativa*) is widely used for medical purposes. Not just smoked, cannabis is used for cooking, to make oils and salves, and is placed into bottles and soaked in rum as an essential part of stress-relieving tonics. Though I am not an advocate of non-medicinal use, I do recognize that marijuana has widespread therapeutic qualities utilized in tonics.

Here in North America, there are many highly effective herbs that can be used for stress relief. Licorice root (*Glycyrrhiza glabra*) helps to normalize blood sugar, regulate the function of the adrenal glands, and stimulate the production of relaxing chemicals in the brain. Chamomile (*Matricaria recutita*) is sweet-tasting and widely available and promotes relaxation. It is known to lower the blood pressure and help you to feel relaxed after a stressful day, and even promotes sleep. Lavender (*Lavandula angustifolia*) reduces irritability, and its sweet scent and taste help to promote a widespread feeling of wellness, relaxing the mind and body. St. John's wort (*Hypericum perforatum*) is useful for relief from depression, sadness, and seasonal affective disorder (SAD). It has a natural anti-anxiety effect and relieves stress. Valerian (*Valeriana officinalis*) is known for promoting sleep and a deep state of restfulness, and is a mild sedative that is useful for relieving shock and anxiety. Indian ginseng (*Withania somnifera*), also known as ashwagandha, helps to regulate the production of cortisol, and combats stress on a cellular level.

For stress relief, use equal parts of valerian rhizome, licorice root, Siberian ginseng root (*Eleutherococcus senticosus*), and kava root (*Piper methysticum*).

To promote sleep, consider making a tonic from equal parts of valerian, chamomile, and lavender.

Make an energy tonic with American ginseng (*Panax quinquefolius*) or Chinese ginseng (*Panax ginseng*), rosemary (*Rosmarinus officinalis*), gotu kola (*Centella asiatica*), and sage (*Salvia* spp.).

Memory Tonics

Many herbs are used as memory tonics. Common herbs used to support healthy brain function, improved memory, and focused concentration include sage (*Salvia officinalis*), skullcap (*Scutellaria lateriflora*), gingko leaf (*Gingko biloba*), gotu kola (*Centella asiatica*), and rosemary (*Rosmarinus officinalis*). Both gotu kola and gingko leaf strengthen the memory, and stimulate cerebral circulation, taking oxygen to the brain cells, which in turn improves their health and function.

Peppermint and rosemary improve memory when used in aromatherapy. Their scents help stimulate memory recall, improving both speed and accuracy. Sage has been shown to improve the communication between different lobes of the brain, boosting interconnectivity and high-level executive thinking.

A simple recipe for making a brain tonic consists of combining 4 parts gotu kola, 4 parts gingko leaf, 2 parts peppermint, 1 part rosemary, and 1 part sage.

Because brain tonics are best used over a long period of time (three to six months), why not make a huge batch to last you? And if you have a huge amount sitting around, you just might remember to take it. Working on a profoundly energetic level, herbal tonics take a longer period to reach "therapeutic" levels within the body. Consider three months as a good length of time to take a tonic.

Making Alcohol-Based Tonics

As with marijuana, I am not a big fan of alcohol either. But, while I am an abstainer, I use alcohol in the production of therapeutic remedies. It is a reliable preservative and carrier for the healing qualities of herbs. Many people use a generic form of grain alcohol, but using wine, brandy, or vodka is also commonplace.

While we can make therapeutic remedies for minor ailments ourselves, it is recommended that you seek out the expertise and assistance of a trained herbalist to help you address chronic ailments or acute disease. A knowledgeable herbalist will help diagnose your ailment and prescribe the herbs most suited to remedy it. Once armed with a diagnosis and prescription, you can successfully and easily make your own tonics to bring your system back to balance.

Follow these steps to make a wide variety of herbal tonics at home:

1. Choose the kind of alcohol you prefer.

2. Place all of the herbs, in correct ratio according to the recipe, in a jar.

3. Cover with alcohol, ensuring there is no air remaining in the jar when it is sealed. The presence of air can allow mold to develop.

4. Seal the jar, and place it in a dark location away from direct sunlight, which can also stimulate mold development. In Jamaica, it is traditional to bury the jar underground.

5. Allow the tonic to steep for six to eight weeks.

6. When decanting, use a fine sieve or cheesecloth to strain out the herbal matter.

7. Store tonic in a clean glass bottle.

8. Label with the name of the tonic, a list of ingredients, and the date it was made.

Back to Balance

Always store your tonic away from direct sunlight and at a cool temperature. Tonics have a long shelf life because of the alcohol content but require occasional agitation to keep sediments from forming, and should be discarded after a year.

Alcohol-based tonics can be consumed on their own or diluted in water or tea. Wine tonics are tasty and make nice after-meal aperitifs. It is best to consume herbal tonics three times a day for a period of at least three months in order to attain maximum benefit.

Now, sip your tonic, and as the warm spread of alcohol affects your throat, know that the healing quality of the herbs is also spreading into your body, helping you to come back to balance.

Dallas Jennifer Cobb *practices gratitude magic, giving thanks for personal happiness, health, and prosperity; meaningful, rewarding, and flexible work; and a deliciously joyful life. She is accomplishing her deepest desires. She lives in paradise with her daughter in a waterfront village in rural Ontario, where she regularly swims and runs, chanting: "Thank you, thank you, thank you." Contact her at jennifer.cobb@live.com.*

The Kitchen Pharmacy

❧ By Autumn Damiana ❧

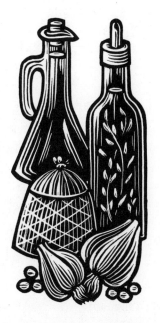

People interested in herbal healing and home remedies are probably familiar with old standbys such as prunes for constipation or chicken soup for the flu, but did you know there are many other staple foods you have in your kitchen right now that can also be used to cure common ailments? Sometimes we forget that food can be medicine, too, and that using food in this manner is one of the cheapest, easiest, and most accessible ways to heal. (Note: The information presented here is for educational purposes only and should not replace the advice of a licensed medical practitioner.)

Powerhouse Cures

Look in your fridge, spice cabinet, and pantry. Although there are various foods that could be considered essential in the kitchen pharmacy, I feel that the following four deserve special mention, since each one seems to have quite a large and dedicated following in the natural health world.

Cider Vinegar

Sometimes I think that there is nothing this won't cure! Drinking just a few tablespoons of raw, unfiltered, unpasteurized cider vinegar in water daily will boost the immune system, break down foods for digestion, detoxify the body, and speed up metabolism. It can be used on skin and hair to restore pH balance, improving both appearance and texture. To cure a sore throat, gargle with a little cider vinegar in which minced garlic has been steeped with a pinch of salt, or add a few tablespoons to a half gallon of water for an odor-neutralizing foot soak.

Honey

Eating locally produced honey daily can help immunize against seasonal allergies, since the honey is likely made from the same local pollen causing the allergic reaction. Honey has also long been known to have antibacterial and antiseptic properties due to its natural imperishability, and can be used to disinfect wounds and seal them against bacteria and possible infection. For this reason, it can also help clear up acne. Honey is also beneficial when drunk in medicinal teas (see recipes later in this article).

Olive Oil

This "liquid gold" is not only a healthy fat for cooking but is also an excellent skin treatment. Use it on scalds and burns to relieve pain and reduce blistering and scarring. Olive oil absorbs easily and can be used as a natural moisturizer for hair, skin, chapped lips, and dry or brittle nails. It also makes an excellent massage oil to ease headaches, backaches, bruises, sprains, and joint or muscle soreness. In addition, a few drops of warmed olive oil inside the ear will relieve an earache, and consuming two tablespoons olive oil daily is effective against constipation.

Garlic

This potent bulb, dubbed "the stinking rose," is already renowned for its cardiovascular health benefits. However, it is also a wonderful antimicrobial and antiviral, and the juice can be used to disinfect cuts and scrapes and is said to work wonders on cold sores. Eating garlic regularly helps ward off colds and flu and discourages biting insects. However, the best use I've found for garlic is as a treatment for yeast infections. Because a sealed garlic clove is sterile inside its papery husk, all you need to do is peel the garlic and place the clove inside the vagina, changing every few hours for three to five days or longer as needed. You can also wrap the garlic in cheesecloth and tie it with unwaxed dental floss to make a kind of tampon for easy extraction. I know this sounds strange, but it really does work!

Quick Kitchen Fixes

The following is a list of simple remedies to reach for in a hurry, especially if you don't have the time, money, or means to go to the drugstore or you can't see the doctor or dentist right away.

- For instant fresh breath, chew parsley or mint leaves. Chewing fennel, dill, or anise seeds will also cleanse the mouth and eliminate burping.

- Drinking cranberry juice is effective in fighting urinary tract or bladder infections. Choose only unsweetened juice, and dilute in up to 3 to 4 parts water to taste.

- Eat a banana with honey to cure hangovers. Bananas are also useful as a natural antacid or to treat muscle cramps and spasms.

- Baking soda paste, made with water or cider vinegar, can be smeared on bug bites to ease the itch. When brushed on teeth, this same paste will act as a natural tooth whitener.

- Women who suffer from PMS or other hormonal imbalances can correct these issues by drinking pomegranate juice.

- Developed for children, the BRAT diet (bananas, rice, applesauce, and toast) is also handy for treating diarrhea and stomach flu in adults.

- Put ½ to ¾ cup oatmeal in muslin or cheesecloth. Tie it closed and add to bathwater to soothe dry skin or the all-over itch from sunburn, rashes, hives, or poison ivy / oak.

- Yogurt with live active cultures used topically on yeast infections, jock itch, and athlete's foot will help kill the infection as well as relieve the symptoms. It doesn't hurt to eat some yogurt for further treatment, either.

A Brief Look at Teas

Entire books have been written on the healing properties of tea. While herbal teas are not "tea" in the strictest sense, they are prepared and consumed in the same way. To make an herbal tea, the common consensus is to use 2 tablespoons roughly chopped or crushed fresh herb (root, spice, flower, etc.) or 1 tablespoon dried herb for 8 ounces (1 cup) water. Purists will recommend that you boil your water separately and then brew your tea in a preheated clay or ceramic vessel with a lid (such as a teapot) and that you add an extra spoonful of herbs when making an entire batch of tea. However, to make just one serving, simply warm your cup (or mug) under a hot tap, add the herbs and water, and then steep the tea in the cup with a plate over the top to hold the heat in. For best results, use a tea infuser instead of tea bags, and don't steep longer than 5 to 10 minutes. For a stronger tea, use more herbs, not a longer brew time. And don't be afraid to flavor your tea the healthy way, with honey, agave nectar, stevia, lemon, or a drop or two of vanilla or almond extract.

Cinnamon Tea

Dissolve 1 teaspoon ground cinnamon and 1 to 2 tablespoons honey per cup (or whole cinnamon sticks can be broken up and used with the previous basic recipe). This powerful combination is said to have healing effects on arthritis, high cholesterol, cold and flu symptoms, and stomach and digestive issues, and it even works for weight loss and regulating blood sugar levels.

Mint Tea

This tea will calm an upset stomach and reduce queasiness, facilitate digestion, ease heartburn, and treat a variety of intestinal issues, including diarrhea, gas, and irritable bowel syndrome. It is also useful for soothing coughs and congestion, and can even help prevent you from getting sick. I like to have a cup before bedtime to ease a headache, relax the nerves, or lull me into a peaceful sleep.

Ginger Tea

Although ginger has many of the same uses as mint and is also famous for treating stomach ailments and nausea (especially caused by motion sickness), ginger tea has a few of its own uses, too. Its anti-inflammatory properties make it useful for easing sore muscles and joints and relaxing cramps and spasms, especially menstrual cramps. Ginger tea will also increase circulation.

Lemon Tea

Try 1 tablespoon lemon juice with 2 tablespoons sugar or honey per cup, flavored with cinnamon, clove, allspice, etc., to alleviate cold and flu symptoms or to get a good dose of vitamin C. For a stubborn cough or to make you sleepy, add a shot of whiskey or other liquor and enjoy a classic hot toddy!

These ideas are just a glimpse into the world of the kitchen pharmacy. It is my hope that in writing this, I have sparked your interest in the idea of using your own kitchen as a pharmacy, and that you will do your own research and see what other food medicines you can discover. Here's to your health!

Autumn Damiana *is passionate about teaching, eco-friendly living, nature, art, and spirituality, and she writes about these and other musings in her blog* Sacred Survival in a Mundane World *at autumn damiana.blogspot.com. She is also an avid crafter, and in her spare time creates pieces for her Etsy store at www.etsy.com/shop/Autumn Damiana. Contact her at autumdamiana@gmail.com.*

The Guardians:
Elder, Hawthorn, and Birch

⤞ By Calantirniel ⤝

This trio of herbs is called the "Guardians" by Philip and Stephanie Carr-Gomm in *The Druid Plant Oracle,* due to the plants' synergistic immune-building qualities. While the Carr-Gomms' work explores the lore and divinatory qualities of these trees, this article instead more deeply explores the healing and medicinal actions, alone and in a group.

Elder
(Sambucus nigra ssp. *canadensis)*

An ancient staple tree medicine used by the Europeans as well as the Native Americans, elder flowers and berries

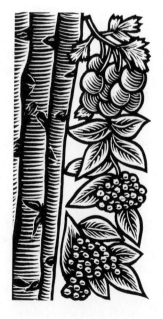

open all of the tubes of the body for slow yet deep and powerful healing and release. This quality also makes the herb quite versatile; it is used to treat respiratory blockage, lymph drainage, kidney/bladder problems, irregular menstruation, and even uterine fibroids. Skin conditions like weepy eczema, poison ivy rash, and even ringworm are curtailed. Elder can also be used for those with either a reddish or bluish cast to their skin, which shows its versatility in feverish and chilly conditions.

The white flowers and blue-black berries, being the safest parts to use, are expectorant, demulcent, diaphoretic, antispasmodic, diuretic, emetic, and oddly stimulant and sedative simultaneously, the effect of which is a normalizing action. Stronger and possibly toxic parts if overused are the antifungal young leaves, and the laxative, purgative bark. Use some fresh or dried berries or alternatively a small amount of dried elder flowers (mixed with other milder herbs—peppermint is a good example) for colds, fever, cough, flu-like symptoms, and even croup or pneumonia. Make and drink a hot strong tea a few times a day for wellness in a short time. The berries also are often prepared in wines, syrups, cordials, or elixirs and have a pleasant taste. The fresh white flowers make a wonderful tea, whereas the dried flowers are stronger tasting.

Known as the "Elder Mother," this tree is said to haunt whomever wishes to cut it down. Despite elder's excellent medicine for infants, it was considered dangerous for a baby to sleep under this tree for fear of a changeling taking its place.

Hawthorn
(*Crataegus* spp.)

If there were ever an herb that would be deemed heart food or heart medicine, it would be hawthorn. Although a relative new-comer as European medicine, having a longer history in Arabic medicine, it has become most important to build, strengthen, restore, and balance the heart and circulatory system and is deemed the supreme cardiac tonic. Matthew Wood, author of *The Earthwise Herbal,* notes that the flavonoid rutin is believed to reduce wear and tear on the capillaries, which would im-prove blood circulation and remove heat congestion. It is also noted for raising HDL cholesterol while lowering LDL choles-terol, bringing a normalizing effect, and is especially helpful with high (or low) blood pressure. Interestingly, there are case studies of rutin showing amazing improvement with autoim-mune disorders and great promise for the treatment of autism, even in one-drop doses of the tincture (preferably of the ber-ries in brandy). Hawthorn berries can also be dried, ground, and made as tea, or you may be able to locate a jam or jelly to embrace these health benefits.

Hawthorn in lore is well reputed to be a fairy tree, and the flowers were usually integrated in the May Queen's crown for the fertility celebration of Beltane, or May Day. In this trio, where elder is noted as the "mother," hawthorn is more like a "father," bringing its wonderfully tonic nutritional support to our very life blood.

Birch
(Betula alba, Betula lenta)

The cool, refreshing wintergreen aroma of birch can give us clues to its healing powers. The leaves, bark, and sap are used in medicine, which was better understood by the Scandinavians. Traditional use in Germany includes drinking the hot tea made of leaves or using the sap in the spring to help detoxify the blood, muscles, and joints, removing protein and mineral waste from heavy winter diets. Birch's diuretic quality will not inflame the kidneys when removing these waste products, and these qualities are emphasized when the tea is brewed and cooled. The cleansing joint and muscle action is most helpful with arthritis, gout, and fibromyalgia. Birch can even dissolve mineralized and fatty deposits, including kidney stones (try the fresh buds for gallbladder issues). Its diaphoretic quality is useful with fever treatment when the tea is served hot. It works well to bring circulation in the extremities and helps varicose veins. Due to the bark's appearance as per the doctrine of signatures, it is a great treatment internally and externally for the skin, especially if there are dry or mineralized deposits (sclerosis). A noteworthy use is as a hair tonic, particularly when combined with nettle (*Urtica* spp.) for creating a daily hair rinse—for oily or dry hair. And unlike elder, birch is considered a safe herb, so drink as much of the tea as needed without worry. Interestingly, while varieties of birch grow in North America, it is underutilized as medicine.

Known as the "Lady of the Woods," birch was known to provide protection against evil and witchcraft, and as the most poetic, revered tree in Russia and central Europe, according to

Northern European lore. In this tree trio, birch can also resonate with the energy of the "child" archetype, as it represents
birth and renewal.

The Guardians in Combination

We can recognize the cleansing, balancing, and nutrition-
ally restorative qualities of these three tree medicines, and
they combine well for our healing purposes. They strengthen
the immune system, allowing us to remain vital and healthy
throughout the seasons, especially with weather changes. Matthew Wood shares a case wherein the first two herbs were combined with cherry bark to permanently eliminate the need for
a serious sinus-related surgery for a patient. These three herbs
singly or in any combination can be used when the seasons are
changing (spring and autumn) to sustain our energy and to
provide a firm foundation of health and well-being. May this
herbal trio bring blessings of health and vigor to you!

Resources

Carr-Gomm, Philip and Stephanie. *The Druid Plant Oracle.*
New York: St. Martin's Press, 2007.

Wood, Matthew. *The Earthwise Herbal: A Complete Guide to
Old World Medicinal Plants.* Berkeley, CA: North Atlantic
Books, 2008.

Calantirniel *has been published in nearly two dozen Llewellyn annuals since 2007 and has practiced many forms of natural spirituality for two decades. She is a professional astrologer, herbalist, tarot
card reader, dowser, energy healer, ULC reverend, and flower essence*

creator/practitioner. She recently realized that her most marketable skill is an uncanny sense for precise event timing. After a decade in western Montana raising her children (who are now doing well on their own), she is back in San Diego, California. She is creating a psychic timing membership-subscription e-course website to teach other psychics these skills. She is also a co-founder of Tië eldaliéva, meaning "the Elven Path," a spiritual practice based upon the elves' viewpoint in Tolkien's Middle-Earth stories. Please visit http://astroherbalist.com.

Tea for You

≋ By Sally Cragin ≋

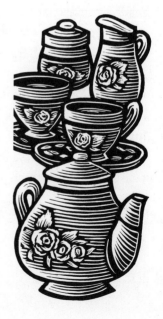

One of the best plays I've seen lately is *Tea for Three*, which my friend Elaine Bromka (Emmy Award–winning actress!) cowrote with Eric H. Weinberger. In this one-woman show, Elaine portrays Lady Bird Johnson, Pat Nixon, and Betty Ford on their last day in the White House. The tradition is that the outgoing First Lady hosts a tea party *a deux* for the new resident. It's a funny and insightful show, and even though Lady Bird would rather be eating chocolate and Betty Ford having a cocktail, it shows how universal, ubiquitous, and downright official the tea party has become.

A proper tea party will have specific accoutrements: a china teapot, loose tea, a bowl with lemon, sugar, and a pitcher of cream. Cups come with saucers, and someone plays "mother"—that is, pours the tea for everyone else. When's the last time you had that experience?

Humans have dried herbs and poured hot water over them and drank them for millenia, but the Western tradition of ingesting teas from the Far East only extends back a few centuries. Tea has prompted civil unrest, like the colonists who hurled three crates overboard in the Boston Tea Party. This act of rebellion helped ignite the American Revolution. Tea parties also provided a surrealistic background for author Lewis Carroll; who can forget the Mad Hatter's absurd tea party? Yes, tea is everywhere, and in my unremarkable downtown grocery store, there are at least twelve horizontal feet of shelf space six feet high devoted to tea boxes—everything from black tea made by gigantic corporations to various herbal concoctions made by smaller vendors.

If you don't know what you're looking for, it's easy to be overwhelmed, so here is some guidance for sampling. And just a note about correctness: proper "tea" is made from the tea plant, *Camellia sinensis*. Herbal drinks are aptly called "infusions" or "decoctions" (if they require boiling). I am sticking to the word "tea" for simplicity's sake. Thanks to Emily French of Sweetgrass Herbals in Sterling, Massachusetts, who assisted in the research process of this article.

Alertness

Are you a caffiend? Then, my friend, you would enjoy teas both black and green. Herbal tea does not have caffeine—unless you're sampling yerba mate or a tea that uses cocoa or chocolate. Less well-known are yerba mate's cousins, guayusa and yaupon. Guarana is another caffeinated plant, related to maple trees and found in the Amazon. Emily recommends thinking about getting energy from "infusions of deeply nourishing plants, including nettle, holy basil, and other adaptogens, such as herbs and mushrooms." For taste, try astragalus root and milky oat tops. When brewing tea with caffeine, I'm always vigilant about the time of infusion, and generally remove the bag after five minutes. You can be much more lenient with other herbs.

Calmness

In my house, chamomile tea is known as "Peter Rabbit tea," because that is, of course, what Mother Rabbit fed him after he limped back from rampaging through Mr. McGregor's garden. It has sleep-aiding properties, and it's also calming. I've found that making tea from dried chamomile flowers—not tea bags—produces a more aromatic, complex taste. I'm curious to grow the plant (Roman and German chamomile are the dominant strains), but until I do, I'm happy making a pot of tea at a time. Other calming plants include passionflower, linden flower, milky oats, and scullcap infusions (mixed or alone). "There's something to be said for the old wisdom of warm milk before bed, so add some to herbal tea if you like," says Emily. "It's wonderfully relaxing."

To make and serve "Peter Rabbit tea," use a heaping tablespoon of dried chamomile flowers for a pot of tea. There's no harm in letting this steep for 15 to 20 minutes, or however long it takes you to drink it. Pour the dregs into a houseplant.

Digestion

The tradition in the West is to follow a meal with coffee and dessert. If you've had a rich dinner, this might be one plate over the line. I'm happy to serve guests what they prefer after dining, but I also have started offering a "digestif" at the very end: a tea with ginger, licorice, and fennel. Ginger tea is easy to find, and if folks think it's too spicy, licorice root will soften the spiciness. You can serve these different herbs in various proportions, but I've sampled a variety and have to recommend a particular brand made by Pukkaherbs.com. Check out their "After Dinner" blend—it has many pleasing notes. Cinnamon is also excellent for digestion. Impress the guests by sprinkling some on your filter coffee before adding hot water.

Immune System

I've noticed over the past few years that holy basil tea, also known as *tulsi* or *tulasi* tea, is getting more popular. Of course, it's not a newcomer, as it's been grown in India for centuries and is one of the plants used in Ayurvedic medicine as an immune-system booster. Tulsi also has anti-inflammatory properties and is said to help you resist stress and to support your eyesight. How much to drink? Anywhere from one to four cups a day. This tea is recommended for those who need help with digestion, suffer with stress-related conditions, or need stamina. Other herbs for helping the immune system are ginger and milky oats. "In the winter, the antibacterial, antiviral, and immune-strengthening properties come in really handy," says Emily. And don't forget turmeric, which has an amazing orange color. This Indian spice is good for inflamed muscles. I'm currently battling Lyme disease and have been drinking turmeric tea, which I make myself (see recipe later in this article). This tea is a very cheerful color!

Female Support

Like it or not, we women are in tune with the moon. If you are feeling familiar aches and twinges in your womb, consider warm tea, and a warm, wet compress on your belly. There are many varieties of herbs that offer support for female bodies, including black cohosh and raspberry leaves. We have raspberry bushes in our yard, and after the harvest, my husband cuts the "runners" (stray vines). These dry quickly, and a handful in a teapot can make an infusion you can drink all day.

If you enjoy foraging, red clover is another good female tonic. Gather the blossoms in summer (avoid plants growing near roadways). Wash, hang in bunches in a shady place, and make a tea with a handful of blossoms and a tablespoon or so of dried mint. The color is pretty, too. Some of these teas have an acquired taste, so if you're serving to guests, make sure they're on board with the purpose. Also, if you're drinking mint or raspberry leaf tea by the pot, you'll get a lot of fluids into your system without sugar or caffeine.

Respiratory Assistance

The germs that prompt coughing come special delivery in wintertime, don't they? If you've taken all your precautions (washed your hands, avoided touching door handles, etc.) and you still feel woozy, consider herbs such as licorice, echinacea, and eucalyptus for relief. If you have the chills, try ginger or cinnamon, which are also great for your immune system. If you're feeling hot and feverish, try a cooling tea like parsley, an herb also known for its anti-inflammatory properties.

Summertime

Only the British make a custom of drinking hot tea in the summertime. For the majority of us colonials, iced tea is the way to go. However, if you're icing black tea, it's easy to get a lot of stimulating caffeine into your system accidentally. I look for decaffeinated black teas (hard to find, but they do exist) or make a tea from either passionflower, blueberry, or raspberry tea bags, with some chamomile mixed in. My favorite summer drink is two bags of chamomile and one bag of peppermint tea in a clear glass quart bottle. Put it out in the morning and let it "cook" in the sun for a couple hours. Chill in the fridge, then serve to guests at dinner. And though this isn't exactly a "tea," you can also jazz up a quart of cold water by adding slices of cucumber and some lime or lemon juice for a refreshing post-exercise beverage.

Wintertime

My favorite warm beverage in the winter is an old Yankee concoction: a tablespoon of apple cider vinegar mixed with honey in hot water. The vinegar and honey boost your immune system, and the hot water opens you up. I learned this from an old-timer decades ago and have sworn by it ever since. If you're battling a cold, go easy on the honey, since bacteria thrives on sweets and sugars. Or try the autumn spice tea recipe given later in this article.

A Few Words about Ayurvedic Teas

Ayurvedic lore and health assistance are definitely trending upward, and I've sampled a few brands of tea with "Ayurvedic" in their titles. My favorite is made by an Iowa company called

Maharishi Ayurveda Products International (mapi.com). Their teas use simple ingredients such as cardamom, cinnamon, licorice, ginger, cloves, pepper, turmeric, and saffron and are tasty and reasonably priced. You may also want to experiment with spices you have in your kitchen with some of the following recipes.

Herbal Tea Recipes

You can make up a batch of tea and store it in a dark glass jar. Add a ribbon and give as a gift along with an infusion spoon. Lemongrass is widely available in Asian markets—remove the woody outer covering and dice the interior stalk. It's very aromatic and keeps well. These recipes will make a pot of tea.

Anise Tea

Grind up 3 large anise stars, or 5 small ones, with a mortar and pestle. Add 1 tablespoon of chamomile flowers or 2 chamomile tea bags. Infuse for at least 7 minutes.

Gingermint Tea

Take a piece of ginger the size of your thumb, and peel and slice. Add 1 tablespoon of peppermint. I like to infuse this tea all day—the ginger keeps getting stronger.

Lemongrass Tea

Cut up a stalk of lemongrass and add a pinch of thyme. Sage will also work, or experiment with other spices as long as you don't overwhelm the delicate tang of the lemongrass.

Autumn Spice Tea

As the weather turns colder, you'll want to be warm, inside and out. Try 3 parts anise, 1 part cinnamon, and 1 part cloves.

If you have vanilla, add ½ teaspoon. This tea is spicy, but the flavors blend well.

Turmeric Tea

For 1 cup of tea, mix a pinch of cayenne with a teaspoon of turmeric. Pour boiling water over it, and mix well. There will be some residue as you are drinking; just add more hot water. For a pot of tea, consider designating a cotton bag for the turmeric, as it is a powder.

Sources

DrWeil.com. "Healthy Turmeric Tea." www.drweil.com/drw/u/ART02833/turmeric-tea.

Interview with Emily French, Herbalist at Sweetgrass Herbals in Sterling, Massachusetts.

Wildflower Apothecary. "The Health Benefits of Tulsi Tea." www.wildflowerapothecary.com/the-health-benefits-of-tulsi-tea.

Sally Cragin *is a teacher and the author of* Astrology on the Cusp, *for people whose birthdays are at the end of one sun sign or the beginning of the next. Her first book is* The Astrological Elements. *She has written the astrological forecast "Moon Signs" for the* Boston Phoenix *newspaper chain, syndicated throughout New England. Re-elected to the Fitchburg, MA, School Committee, she is the only professional astrologer holding elected office in New England. She also provides forecasts for clients that are "cool, useful, and accurate." Read more at moonsigns.net or e-mail sallycragin@verizon.net.*

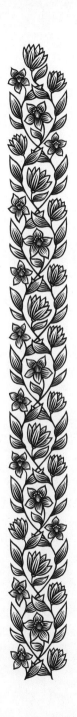

Herb Crafts

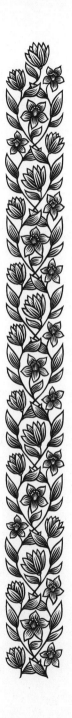

Lovely Lavender Gifts

⇜ By Deborah Castellano ⇝

The smell of crushed lavender is intoxicating. The sweet, rich floral scent ends with a slightly camphorous, pungent citrus smell. There's no other scent like it in the world.

The name lavender actually represents a family of plants, the most common of which are French lavender (*Lavandula dentata*) and English lavender (*Lavendula officinalis*). There are many other kinds of lavender as well, some of which aren't even lavender-colored! Lavender can be found in luscious yellow and cerise red in addition to the more widely known bluish violet. English and French are the best types of lavender for scent and culinary purposes, however.

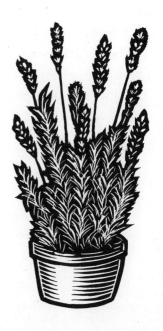

French lavender has a delicate scent with an undertone of rosemary-like notes, whereas English lavender has a more robust aroma. French lavender can be used for scent purposes, such as dried lavender bud sachets or essential oils. English lavender can be used for both its sensual properties and culinary uses.

Lavender has been used for centuries to help with a variety of ailments and is used today in homeopathic medicine to help with issues such as insomnia, anxiety, depression, upset stomach, and headaches.

Lavender Gifts

Lavender's healing properties combine with its popularity as a perfume scent to make the perfect gift for any occasion.

Lavender-Infused Oil

It has taken me some time to perfect my lavender-infused oil. Some people swear by making theirs in a slow cooker, but I've always burned mine there. The most important ingredient in this method is patience!

 1 cup dried lavender buds

 1 ¼ cups grapeseed or almond oil

 1 tablespoon vitamin E oil (to keep the oil from going off)

 Equipment: mortar and pestle, a microwave-safe plastic container and lid, microwave, French press coffeemaker, eyedropper, glass amber bottles, labels (optional)

Fill your mortar about ½ full with the dried lavender buds and dribble in about ⅛ cup of the grapeseed (or almond) oil. Use your pestle to crush the buds into the oil so that they release as much of their fragrance as possible. Mix for about 10 minutes. Pour your mixture into your container along with the rest of the oil and the vitamin E oil. Put the lid on tightly. Shake up your mixture in its container. Microwave for 30 seconds. Keep the mixture in a cool, dark place, remembering to shake it every few days. Every time you shake it, microwave it for 30 seconds. Do this for 2 weeks. Pour your mixture into your French press and use it to press the oil. Wash out the plastic container and then pour the oil back into the container. The oil should now be free of the dried buds and ready to be decanted into your glass bottles with the eyedropper, and labeled if you desire.

Lavender Sugar Body Scrub

Sugar is a great natural exfoliate, and lavender oil can increase blood circulation. Combining the two makes them perfect for exfoliating in the shower. The scrub can be used with a loofah or mesh shower poof. This is a great gift for your bath-product-obsessed loved one.

   1 cup sugar

   1 teaspoon lavender oil (either your infused oil or
      commercial lavender oil)

   ¾ cup grapeseed or almond oil

   Equipment: wooden or plastic mixing spoon, 32-ounce
      container with a lid (such as a Mason jar), mixing bowl,
      label (optional)

Mix the sugar, lavender oil, and grapeseed oil together. Pour into your container and seal the lid. Label if desired.

Lavender Pillow Spray

Nothing is more soothing than the smell of lavender on your pillow after a long day. Lavender pillow spray makes a great gift for a new parent or for anyone who has trouble sleeping. Nighty night!

> 1 milliliter vodka (to help the spray evaporate)
>
> 1 tablespoon lavender oil (either your infused oil or commercial lavender oil)
>
> Distilled water
>
> Equipment: 1 small spray bottle (can be found at a drugstore), eyedropper, label (optional)

Using the eyedropper, pour the vodka into the spray bottle. Add the lavender oil. Fill the bottle the rest of the way with the distilled water. Shake well. Label if desired.

Lavender Felted Soap

Felted soap is a great gift for someone who travels a lot because it packs very nicely. The wool felt acts as a natural loofah, while the goat's milk soap is an amazing moisturizer. The more you use the soap, the more the wool naturally felts. As the soap gets smaller, the felt casing will shrink with it. At the end, you have a naturally biodegradable wool case that will be kind to the earth.

> Melt-and-pour goat's milk soap (available online and in craft stores)
>
> 1 ounce lavender essential oil (commercial or infused)
>
> Dyed wool roving (roving is a narrow, long bundle of fiber—can be purchased on Etsy)

Knee-high stockings

Water

Equipment: silicone soap molds, a double boiler, mixing
   bowl, towels, bamboo sushi rolling mat

Put water into the pot part of your double boiler, then put the
melt-and-pour soap and lavender oil in the bowl part. Set the
heat to medium on your stove. When the soap has melted,
pour it into the molds. Let cool for an hour and then pop the
soap out of the molds. Wrap the soap in roving so that the roving completely covers the soap and none of the soap shows
through. Put the roving-covered soap into the knee-high stocking, and tie the stocking in a knot close to the soap. Run the tap
as hot as it can go, and put the stocking under it for a minute.
Let it cool for a moment and then turn it over in your hands
until you see the soap lather up.

Fill your mixing bowl with very warm water. Put your
bamboo mat on your towels and start running the stocking/
soap over it in all directions—clockwise, counterclockwise, left
to right, right to left, on all sides. Periodically dip the soap in
the water in your mixing bowl and continue rubbing it on your
bamboo mat. Do this for at least 20 minutes per bar of soap.
Run your tap as hot as it will go, and dip your stocking/soap
in it. Then run your tap as cold as it will go and repeat. Do this
a few times; the drastic change in temperature will help your
soap felt better. When you take the stocking off the soap, the
roving should be felted closely to the soap. If it isn't, put it back
in the stocking and rub it on the bamboo mat until it is. Let dry
on a towel overnight.

Lavender Tea

This tea is a great caffeine-free bedtime treat to soothe a loved one into blissful sleep.

- 2 tablespoons dried culinary lavender
- 2 tablespoons dried chamomile
- 2 tablespoons dried mint
- 2 tablespoons dried culinary-grade rose petals
- Equipment: 4-ounce glass Mason jar with lid, tea ball, teacup, teakettle, label (optional)

Mix the dried flowers and herbs together in the Mason jar and seal with the lid. Label the jar if desired. When you're ready to brew, pour some of the tea into the tea ball and boil water in your teakettle. Put the tea ball into the teacup and pour the boiling water over it. Let the tea steep for 5 minutes. Remove the tea ball and enjoy.

Lavender Sugar

Lavender sugar is the perfect complement to your lavender tea. Together in a basket (possibly with some lavender tea bread as well), this makes a delightful gift for the tea lover in your life.

- ¼ cup dried culinary lavender buds
- 1 cup sugar
- Equipment: 12-ounce glass Mason jar with lid, label (optional)

Mix the lavender buds with the sugar in the Mason jar and cover tightly. Label the jar if desired. Let sit for 3 days before using or giving so that the lavender will infuse properly with the sugar.

Lavender Tea Bread

Light, sweet, and airy, this quick bread is very easy to make. It makes a great teacher's gift, or make several for your favorite coworkers.

6 tablespoons 1% milk

⅓ cup low-fat sour cream

1 egg, at room temperature

3 teaspoons honey

8 tablespoons sugar

1 cup white or whole wheat flour

½ teaspoon baking powder

¼ teaspoon baking soda

½ teaspoon salt

2 tablespoons lemon curd

¼ cup dried culinary-grade lavender buds

2 tablespoons poppy seeds (optional)

Equipment: oven, mixing bowl, mixing spoon or electric beater, loaf pan or bread machine

If you are baking this bread in your oven, preheat the oven to 350°F. Mix all the ingredients together in a mixing bowl for about 200 strokes if you're mixing by hand, or for about 2 minutes with an electric beater set to medium. Grease a loaf pan and pour the batter into it. Bake for 25 minutes. Let cool for about a half hour and then gently release the bread from the pan. If using a bread machine, put the ingredients in the order listed into your bread machine. Select small loaf, light crust, and use the quick bread setting.

Lavender Lemon Thyme Cordial

Cordial making offers all the satisfaction of home brewery without the complication of fermentation. As with the lavender infused oil, the most important ingredient in this recipe is patience. This makes a lovely holiday gift for extended family and friends. Obviously, this is meant for people who are legally permitted to drink alcohol.

4 lemons

½ cup water

½ cup sugar

1 small bunch of fresh thyme

4 tablespoons dried culinary-grade lavender

1 quart vodka

Equipment: 1½-quart glass Mason jar with lid, zester, juicer, French press coffeemaker, saucepan

Make sure your Mason jar has been washed in the dishwasher or boiled in water in a saucepan so it's clean to use. Zest the lemons and put the zest into the pot. Juice the lemons and add the juice to the saucepan as well. Add the water, sugar, thyme, and lavender to the saucepan. Heat the pan on low-medium until the sugar is dissolved, stirring occasionally. Pour the mixture, including the thyme and lemon zest, into the jar. Add the vodka until the jar is just about full and screw the lid on tightly. Shake it up. Let sit in a cool, dark place for 10 days, shaking every few days. After that, pour it into your French press and press out the herbs and peels, then pour back into your Mason jar. Keep in the refrigerator for up to a week. The finished cordial can be enjoyed alone in a small cordial glass or mixed with sparkling lemonade.

Herbes de Provence

This mixture of herbs originally referred to the kinds of herbs that commonly grow in the Provence region of France. It was only in the 1970s that the company now known as McCormick decided to mix them together to offer as an herbal mixture. The following mix is not actually used in traditional French cooking; it's the American version of this mixture that includes lavender. This mix is great for flavoring meat, soups, and stews and can also be used as popcorn seasoning and baked in with bread. For those watching their sodium content, it's a great way to spice up food without adding salt. This mix makes a great savory gift for your foodie friends.

1 tablespoon culinary-grade dried lavender buds

2 tablespoons dried thyme

2 tablespoons dried marjoram

2 tablespoons dried savory

1 tablespoon dried basil

1 tablespoon dried rosemary

1 teaspoon dried sage

1 teaspoon fennel seeds

Equipment: 6-ounce container (such as a glass Mason jar) with a lid, label (optional)

Mix all the ingredients together. Pour into the container and put the lid on tightly. Label the jar if desired. It will keep fresh for 6 months.

Bibliography

Culpeper, Nicholas. *Culpeper's Complete Herbal*. Wordsworth Editions, 2007.

Green, James. *The Herbal Medicine-Maker's Handbook: A Home Manual*. Crossing Press, 2000.

Grieve, Mrs. M. *A Modern Herbal*. Dorset Press, 1992.

Tierra, Michael. *The Way of Herbs*. Pocket Books, 1998.

Deborah Castellano *enjoys writing about earth-based topics, though she has been known to write romantic fiction as well. Her craft shop, La Sirene et Le Corbeau, specializes in handspun yarn and other goodies. She resides in New Jersey with her husband, Jow, and two cats. She has a terrible reality television habit she can't shake and likes St. Germain liqueur, record players, and typewriters. Visit her at www.deborahmcastellano.com.*

The Fascination of Floral Design: Arrangements with Herbs & Flowers from Your Own Garden

⤜ By Ellen Dugan ⤛

The best thing about growing your own flowers, blooming shrubs, and flowering herbs in the home garden is that it gives you supplies for all sorts of goodies. You may use your herbs for strictly ornamental reasons, to flavor dishes, or for their fragrance and sense of history in the landscape. Or perhaps you prefer to use your herbs for all of the above—plus putting those herbs to work for a bit of enchantment.

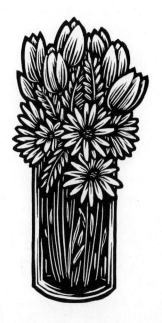

Herbs add a touch of mystery and magic to any garden. However, in my opinion, one of the best things about gardening is that it gives you supplies for floral design for about ten months out of the year.

When I was pregnant with my youngest child, I took an accredited floral design class. At the time (twenty-six years ago), it was the only floral design class available in my area. I waddled in with my boxes of supplies, and over the next six weeks, I learned all sorts of diverse ways to work with silk flowers. We only did one session working with fresh flowers, but the instructor assured me that the mechanics were the same. With my certificate in hand, I strolled out of that class and nabbed a seasonal job working for a local floral designer a few weeks before Thanksgiving.

Talk about your crash course in fresh flowers! The owner was a tough lady who brooked no nonsense from her employees. I impressed her because, even hugely pregnant, I always showed up and worked hard, and best of all, I was a fast learner. Thus my love affair with fresh flowers and floral design began.

A few years later, when my children were older, I was bitten by the gardening bug, which I believe to be just a different sort of floral design. Instead of working in a vase, you are actually arranging the flowers, trees, and shrubs in the ground. The whole landscape becomes a permanent arrangement.

As my gardens matured, I planted with an eye for plants that would bloom almost year round. I made notes of what bloomed and when, ensuring that all year long there would be something in my gardens for me to arrange with. These floral supplies included blooming shrubs, bulbs, herbs, annuals, perennials, biennials, and foliage from evergreens and deciduous trees.

Working in flower shops has taught me that sometimes the best and most interesting fillers are the unexpected ones from nature, including foliage, twisty bare branches, and evergreens.

So with that thought in mind, here are some floral arrangements you can make yourself at home. You can plan on spending anywhere from ten minutes to an hour designing them. It will all depend on your level of experience, your eye for design, and how complicated you wish to make your arrangement.

Keep in mind that these projects are supposed to be fun! So no stressing about it. Go artsy! Go funky with your arrangements! The flowers do not have to be perfectly symmetrical (unless you want them to be). Remember that elements of form, line, and texture are important, but if a bit of something unexpected is in the arrangement, it takes a pedestrian design to the next level of creativity and cleverness. The following directions list florals for spring arrangements. However, there are more seasonal flower suggestions included later in the article. No matter what the season, the design directions stay the same.

Artsy Spring-Blooming Branch Arrangement

Supplies:

- A wide-mouthed vase or old canning jar. (Old Mason jars look both casual and cool and are easy to work in!)

- Fresh water for the container.

- Knife, garden snips, or strong craft scissors.

- A hammer. (Yes, a hammer—you will need it to smash the ends of the branches so they can drink more water.)

- Flowers from your garden. (Spring flowers to consider: tulips, bleeding heart, columbine, daisy, peonies, pansies.)

- Blooming spring branches from the garden. (Consider forsythia, snowball bush, Korean spice viburnum, sand cherry, cherry, dogwood, crab apple, pussy willow.)

- Foliage from the garden. (Consider bleeding heart foliage, violet leaves, peony leaves and stems, young fern fronds.)

- A secure, firm base on which to mash the ends of those branch stems. (Old cutting boards are great.)

- Paper towels and a garbage bag for clean up. (Be prepared for a mess—floral design is not a tidy process.)

No matter what season you are arranging in, gather your flowers and foliage in the morning. If you are not arranging until the afternoon, put the floral material in the refrigerator in a bucket of clean water. (Plant material tends to be full of moisture just after sunrise, so it's the best time to gather for arrangements.) Be sure to strip any foliage—that will be stored in the fridge for later—below the water line. All you want in the storage bucket's water is stems, not leaves or blossoms.

Please be sure to gather the plant material carefully and with consideration. Take the smallest amount possible so you do not harm the plant. A good rule of thumb to follow is to take no more than a fourth of a small plant—a short branch or two from a small shrub, and so on.

Cut or prune the stems and branches cleanly and correctly. Typically, a correct cut on a shrub/tree is just above the next stem/branch junction. Also do NOT raid the park or your neighbor's gardens for supplies! Talk about bad manners.

Floral Design Tip #1

Odd numbers *always* look better in an arrangement. So if you are working with blooming viburnum branches, then use three or five branches instead of two or four. Same goes with the main flowers in your design. Go for an odd number—it's more pleasing to the eye.

Floral Design Tip #2

Start with the blooming branches to build your frame. And again, remember to be sure to strip any foliage or blossoms from the bottom of the branches. All that should be below the water line is the stem. Arrange the branches first. (See the next tip for measuring advice.)

Floral Design Tip #3

A quick way to measure the length of where to cut the stems on the first try is to move the container to the edge of the counter or work surface. Hold the stems up in front of the vase, and then move them up and down to the desired height.

Now, eyeballing it, "mark" where the end of those branches would rest in that vase—which is the edge of the counter. Get it? (By holding the stems right in front of the vase or container, the vase bottom is in fact the top edge of the counter—you can tell exactly how long to cut your stems!) Now snip the stems to the desired length.

Floral Design Tip #4

When in doubt, go long. You can always trim the stems down to a shorter length, but once they are cut too short, that's it. Or you have to use a shorter vase.

Floral Design Reality: Smashing, Stripping, and Arranging Floral Components

Now it's time to smash, strip, and arrange. Sounds brutal, doesn't it? Hey, floral design is not a neat and tidy process. After the woody branches are snipped to the correct length, lay the ends onto an old cutting board and give them a quick rap with a hammer. By smashing the ends of the woody branches, you are allowing more surface area for the blooming branches to drink through. (Winter evergreens such as pine, spruce, and cypress do NOT need to be smashed. They are long-lived and do fine with a fresh, clean cut. Holly, boxwood, and tough ivy stems would benefit from a little smash.)

To begin the arrangement, place the blooming branches in the vase or container. Doing this first builds a sort of frame. This will also help to support the new, additional flower stems.

Next, add the largest flowers to your design. Cut the flower stems on a sharp angle—this also allows for a greater surface area for the flower to draw water through.

If you are working with roses, you may choose to cut off the thorns with a pocket knife before you arrange them. Cut the thorns away by working from the bottom of the stem, and up and away from yourself. The end of the stem will be toward your chest, and the sharp edge of the knife will cut up and away. Cut or shave the thorns off one by one. Be careful, and take your time. I often hold the rose stem over a paper towel when I am stripping thorns, so I can see those fallen thorns as I cut them off—fewer nasty surprises that way when you go to clean up! After you have removed the thorns, measure and cut the rose stem. Add it immediately to the water.

Next, add the medium-size flowers, and so on until you get to the smallest flowers or fillers, such as bleeding heart foliage, feverfew blossoms, or ferns. Adjust the arrangement as you go, but don't pick it to death! Think artsy and casual, not regimented and fussy.

More Ideas and Flower Suggestions for Seasonal Arrangements

The directions for all floral designs are essentially the same. The difference is the seasonal floral components that you gather from your garden. You can always supplement with a few stems of daisies or mums from the local florist if you need to.

Summer Arrangements

Consider working with yarrow, lavender, roses, lamb's ear, blooming sage, baptisia (false indigo), hosta blossoms, day lilies, balloon flowers, foxglove, tall garden phlox, Joe-Pye weed, verbena, and feverfew blossoms. For blooming branches, think butterfly bushes and hydrangea blossoms and foliage. Also look to your ferns and some colorful hosta leaves to add texture to the arrangements.

Autumn Arrangements

Use chrysanthemums, of course! Autumn joy sedum is fabulous as well. Don't forget that roses tend to make a last big push in the autumn. I work with goldenrod, ornamental grasses, monk's hood, pineapple sage, marigolds, zinnias, wild ageratum, rosemary stems, and obedient plant, as well as branches of fragrant sumac, burning bush, and the yellow leaves and stems from the now-faded balloon flower. Look for twisty fallen stems and slim, small branches from colorful deciduous trees. One autumn design idea is to hollow out a medium-sized pumpkin as if you were going to carve a jack o' lantern, and cut the opening large enough to slip a glass jar inside. Now arrange your autumn flowers inside of the vase/pumpkin!

Winter Holiday Arrangements

Use holly branches, green and variegated ivy to trail over the sides of the container, boxwood clippings, rosemary, sage, and pinecones (of course!), as well as pine, cypress, and spruce branches. Attach the pinecones with a twisty tie or floral wire to a small, straightish branch, and tuck into your arrangement. Texture is everything in a winter design.

You may wish to pick up a few red or white stems of mums, carnations, or roses from the local florist if you live in a non-tropical climate. But remember that the majority of the components in professional winter designs are greenery. You can always add a few colorful glass ornaments to a design of a variety of fragrant evergreen. Variegated holly and its red berries would pop against that! Add a sparkly bow, and you have an instant holiday centerpiece.

I hope you have gained a lot of ideas and are inspired to try your hand at floral design. No matter what the season, look to the supplies in your own garden and yard first. Happy arranging!

Ellen Dugan *is an award-winning author and psychic-clairvoyant. She is the author of many Llewellyn books, including her newest titles:* Seasons of Witchery, Witches Tarot, *and* Practical Prosperity Magick. *Ellen wholeheartedly encourages folks to go outside and get their hands dirty, so they can discover the wonder and magick of the natural world. Ellen and her family live in Missouri. Visit her popular syndicated blog at www.ellendugan.blogspot.com. Visit her website at www.ellendugan.com.*

Creating and Owning Your Own Herb Shop

By Clea Danaan

E ver dreamed of owning your own herb shop? I interviewed Tonja Reichley, founder and owner of MoonDance Botanicals in Denver, Colorado, to learn more about creating and managing an herbal apothecary. We also talked about Ireland and fairy magic a little, as she was in Ireland when we chatted via e-mail.

Established in 2002, MoonDance handcrafts all their products with attention and care. The heart of the store is a great wooden century-old apothecary bar lined with big glass jars of herbs, where the shop employees mix herbal elixirs. These healthy "sodas" are a blend of therapeutic herbal tinctures, infused herbal honeys, and

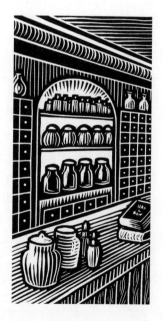

flower hydrosols, designed to both refresh and heal. One can also purchase fresh face masks made from sumptuous ingredients like pumpkin, dark chocolate, and rose water. The shop's shelves are stocked with handmade herbal soaps, beauty products, and salves, as well as jewelry, clothing, and cards made by local artisans. They even carry locally made, high-quality hula-hoops!

In the store's intimate and peaceful classroom space, one can participate in spa parties, classes, and fairy-themed birthday parties. MoonDance also offers massage, Reiki, and tarot readings. The whole space feels protected by the herbs, stones, and gifts that fill the shop. On a warm day, with the door open, you can smell the delicious aroma of the store as you pass by on the street. Upon entering through the bright red door, your tensions seem to melt a little as your spine straightens. You can feel how this is a place of respect, magic, healing, and power.

I interviewed Tonja via e-mail about what it is like to own and manage such a unique business. We e-mailed back and forth several times while she was in Ireland on retreat and I was in Denver. I have edited our chats for clarity and flow.

Clea Danaan: Please tell me a little about your shop and how it is run.

Tonja Reichley: MoonDance Botanicals is an herb shop in a general sense, although in addition to bulk herbs, custom teas, and other herbal remedies, we handcraft over 150 all-natural products for body, mind, and spirit. Set up in the artisanal European tradition, we handcraft all of our products in small batches right in the shop so customers can observe their products being made daily.

Our shop community includes shop ladies (and men) who self-manage. We operate as a collaborative rather than the usual hierarchical scheme so common in America. Everyone who works at MoonDance has extensive herbal experience and has interned at the shop for at least three months. In addition to our shop ladies (managers), we have an internship program that is vital to our community. Interns commit to being at the shop one day per week for three months to learn herbal crafting and deepen their working knowledge of herbs.

Clea Danaan: Besides being at the shop once a week, what do interns do to learn the trade?

Tonja Reichley: They take classes at MoonDance and with other herbalists, spend time with the herbs and in the elements, read and learn on their own by experimenting, etc. One of the great things about the internship program is that it teaches them the basic skills needed to really get creative with the herbs. And working with the herbs themselves, whether it be in a plant spirit meditation, in a tea, or using them in a product, is the best way to learn.

Clea Danaan: What motivated you to open an herb shop?

Tonja Reichley: I worked in the corporate world for almost ten years and felt the soullessness of that work. I really felt drawn to find a vocation that mattered to me and, thus, to my world. Back in my corporate days, I found the healing power of herbs and aromatherapy to be profound.

Clea Danaan: I love that you run your shop as a collaborative. In what ways has that been challenging?

Tonja Reichley: One challenge is finding the right sort of person to be able to take ownership of all aspects of running the shop. They need to be able to delegate, make decisions, and feel empowered. I feel blessed with the people who are involved in our collaborative, because I know it takes a unique individual to be able to step into that role while also being an intuitive herbalist!

Clea Danaan: It obviously pays off, though, for your shop is magical and unique. What has running your shop this way taught you about life?

Tonja Reichley: It has taught me that this is how I want to live all of my life relationships. There is very little, if any, difference between how I run my shop and how I raise my daughter and how I enter into a relationship. Basically, I live my life the way I live my shop life. I want to have a clear sense of my place in the collaborative, yet I endeavor to make room for all types of possibility and empowerment for all parties involved.

Clea Danaan: What advice would you give business owners who strive to create a similar structure but still run a successful business?

Tonja Reichley: Release the need to micromanage. This is a tough one; even when I endeavor not to micromanage, I feel my inner detail manager wanting to take over. Also, believe in your employees, and give them freedom to learn and grow where their passions lie. Communicate your vision clearly so you can trust that they will hold that vision for the business. This final one is one reason why it is important for people to intern and take my longer-term classes.

Clea Danaan: How do you feel that being a woman influences you as a business owner?

Tonja Reichley: Bringing in the feminine characteristics of creating a nurturing and sensual place definitely influences my business, as do my more masculine aspects of having an MBA to support the mundane business aspects.

Clea Danaan: MoonDance has changed some over the years. What have you learned since you first opened?

Tonja Reichley: MoonDance has grown very organically over the years, beginning in a wee shop that was open just fifteen hours per week, with me as its only contributor. Today, she is a living vision that I have had in my heart and mind for years. And I have allowed the business to flower in her own time. This is the biggest lesson: to have faith to hold my vision and the patience to see it happen. I have worked hard and stayed true to my vision.

Clea Danaan: It does take patience to see something unfold. What was your original vision?

Tonja Reichley: To create community—a place where people can come and feel nourished, body and spirit.

Clea Danaan: Your shop has such a magical and powerful energy that is also playful and lovely. What are your influences?

Tonja Reichley: My influences are the herbs themselves, our great wisdom teachers, and Brighid, goddess and saint of Ireland.

Clea Danaan: Who are your wisdom teachers?

Tonja Reichley: John O'Donohue, Rainer Marie Rilke, Carl Jung, Juliette de Baïracli Levy (an herbalist), Margaret Atwood, William Butler Yeats, D. H. Lawrence (I just finished reading *Lady Chatterley's Lover*…totally resonated with my soul).

Clea Danaan: And how do herbs themselves help create your store?

Tonja Reichley: The herbs are the basis of my store and of all of our products. We work with the herbs in their purest forms, believing they are thresholds to the Divine, to remembering, to deeper knowing (or unknowing). I and my shop ladies give gratitude to them every single day, and we honor them with love, enthusiasm, and openness, recognizing the power and magic they hold for us.

Clea Danaan: One of the first things one notices when entering the shop, besides the power and magic of the space, is the big wooden and marble backbar of the front counter. Can you tell me about it?

Tonja Reichley: The building that the shop is in was originally built as an apothecary. As soon as I walked in and saw the backbar, I knew that it was the place for MoonDance. The backbar is the only thing that stayed original. The rest of the place was a wreck, so we rebuilt everything else, including the front counter (in front of the backbar). The backbar is amazing, though, and does give it that ancestral feel a bit. The wood is so rich. I think the marble is from Marble, Colorado, too. I love that we are able to bring it back to its original purpose. We saw some pictures [of the original shop], and "fancy goods" was one of the phrases that appeared on the windows originally, so that is why we chose that particular old-fashioned phrase again on our sign [which reads "MoonDance Botanicals: Local.Fresh.Fancy Goods."]. After it was an apothecary, the store was an art gallery for many years and then a health food shop for maybe twenty or twenty-five years, then a florist, and now MoonDance.

Clea Danaan: I love all the jewelry, clothing, and artwork you offer. How do you choose which products to include from other artisans?

Tonja Reichley: I like to support all local artists. I know how tough it is to hand-make things and I honor the courage it takes to put your heart's work out into the world, so I am pretty easy with artisans. I don't have a strict curator process or anything. I am especially drawn to anything botanical, whether it be jewelry or art or cards. We do have a couple of male artists, although primarily I like to support women.

Clea Danaan: The heart of MoonDance is the handmade herbs that you and your interns make in the shop. In working with the herbs and remedies, do you work with herbal devas or spirits?

Tonja Reichley: I work with the individual plant spirits directly. We love to leave gifts for the devas and the fairies and the protectors of the natural world, although it is the individual plant spirits that we join with most often.

Clea Danaan: Say more about working with a plant spirit directly.

Tonja Reichley: I like to enter into meditation with a plant spirit via intentional ritual, being clear on what I would like to learn from the herb and asking to receive her wisdom. When I move into this meditation, if the plant spirit allows, I actually like to enter her body, moving from the roots, swimming in her chlorophyll, and becoming one with her as I travel through her body. While being one with her, [I am] open to receive whatever knowledge and wisdom she is willing to share.

I also endeavor to recognize each herb and each plant as a unique individual. I talk with them, often verbally and always nonverbally. I share with them how much I adore them. They love being appreciated! So, often, I connect with a plant spirit simply by walking by a plant who wants a bit of attention or to whom I want to give a bit of attention.

Clea Danaan: Tonja, thank you for sharing your stories and wisdom with me. Any final advice you would like to give to people who are drawn to working with herbs?

Tonja Reichley: Spend time with the herbs themselves, listening to them, hearing their call. Find an herbalist you resonate with to be your teacher. For me, having a human herb teacher to help open and support the lessons of the herb plant teacher is the essential combination.

Love your mother the earth, and all of her abundance will be returned to you again and again.

Clea Danaan *lives in Colorado with her two homeschooled children, music therapist husband, and three spoiled cats. Her books, including* Living Earth Devotional, Sacred Land, Voices of the Earth, *and* The Way of the Hen, *weave together themes of ecumenical spirituality, green living, permaculture, and personal growth. Learn more at CleaDanaan.com and on Facebook. Visit MoonDance Botanicals at* http://moondancebotanicals.com.

Herbal Sachets

✺ By Charlie Rainbow Wolf ✺

You might remember the lavender bags that your mother and grandmother had in their drawers or hope chests. Perhaps you even helped tie the dried flower heads in pieces of muslin or gauze to make them. These little sachets of dried herbs have been used with linens and for many other uses for a long time.

Potpourris and little bags filled with scented dried herbs and flowers are a wonderful trip back into yesteryear. Clothing drawers are not the only place in which they make welcome additions. They can be placed on closet shelves, hung from clothes rails, and added to storage units and cabinets, as well as tucked into pillows. Little pomanders can also be worn about the

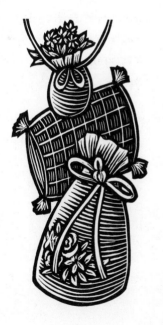

person—they have been used this way throughout history to help protect the wearer from disease, curses, and other dangers. These sachets can be purchased at quite a hefty price from boutiques and specialty shops, but many of the commercial blends contain synthetic oils and perfumes, and these may not be desirable. With a bit of thought and creativity, homemade blends can be created—blends that are completely natural and that often cost much less than their purchased counterparts.

Before starting to gather herbs, decide on how the sachet is going to be used. Herbs that are going to be placed where clothing is kept will probably be different than those added to a cupboard of dishes or placed in a bed pillow. A bit of research will soon reveal which herbs are most suitable for different places.

Cedar is a tree that belongs to several evergreen families, and it makes a great inclusion in herbal sachets that are going to be used where clothing and linens are kept. The use of cedar goes back thousands of years, and the Egyptians used it during mummification. Cedar is a strong insect repellent, which is why so many old linen boxes were made of some kind of cedar wood. Dried cedar can be purchased from most apothecaries and herbal shops. For an added aroma in a household sachet, a few drops of pure essential oil of cedar can be added to the dried cedar—but be careful not to use this where the oil might stain.

Lavender (*Lavandula*) is another favorite for herbal sachets. It is a shrubby plant that is easily grown in herb gardens in all but the most extreme climates. It is the dried flowers that are used when making herbal sachets. Dried lavender can also be purchased easily and inexpensively. This is another wonderful herb that can be added to a blend to keep away moths and other unwanted pests. Like cedar oil, lavender oil may be added for extra scent for use in drawers and cupboards.

Rose petals can easily be dried to use in a sachet. There are many varieties of rose, but my favorite is the *Rosa rugosa*, the old-fashioned rose hip. Pick the newly opened flowers early in the morning, when the dew is off them but the heat of the day has not peaked. Remove the petals from the stem and place them in a warm oven on a very gentle heat, or use a dehydrator on a very low setting if one is available. If purchasing dried rose petals, make sure that they have not been synthetically treated; rose oil is incredibly expensive! Rose petals make a romantic addition to a sachet that is going to be placed in a bed pillow.

Dried hops (*Humulus lupulus*) are a great addition to a sachet that is going to be placed inside a bed pillowcase. Hops have been a common ingredient in beers for about the last five hundred years, but history suggests that they have been used in herbal medicines and in other ways long before brewers found them to be a stabilizing and flavorful additive to the ale. The scent of hops is soothing and mildly sedative. Dried hops can be purchased from herbal stores and home-brewing shops. Ensure that sweet hops rather than bitter hops are obtained for use in this instance.

Other herbs that are suitable for sachets are lilac (*Syringa chinensis*), which is sweet and sensual; lemon balm (*Melissa officinalis*), which combines well with the herbs mentioned previously; mint (*Mentha*), which adds a stimulating aroma; and thyme (*Thymus*), which adds a peaceful note to the blend.

There are some herbs that should be avoided. Rue (*Ruta graveolens*), for example, could make a sleeping sachet too harsh, and great care must be taken in handling rue, as it can cause skin blisters. Good results for different purposes can be reliably achieved, provided a bit of research is done. As always, safety comes first. Ensure that the herbs you use are going to be appropriate for the place and the recipient, as some herbs that seem on the surface to be wonderful inclusions may prove to be inappropriate where there are pets or children who might get hold of the sachets.

After the intention for the sachet is determined and the appropriate herbs are gathered, a suitable pouch in which to put the herbs needs to be either made or obtained. Natural fibers such as wool, cotton, or silk are preferable to humanmade equivalents. They breathe better and allow the aromas of the dried herbs to be dispersed more effectively. Remember that the dried herbs are likely to crumble as they age, so the bag into which they are placed needs to accommodate this.

A good method of providing the herbs with a decorative outer covering and an efficiently protective inner one is to line a more ornate bag with a small muslin or cheesecloth liner. Muslin bags can easily be purchased from craft shops or in bulk from online suppliers. They are inexpensive and provide a good liner for a more ornate exterior. Seamstresses will be able to make these liners with ease, too. If the sachet is just going to be placed in a drawer or cupboard for personal use, this may be all the protection that is needed. If the sachet is going to be given as a gift, a prettier outside may be desired.

The exterior of the pouch is where your creativity can shine. Being an avid knitter, I tend to knit lacy bags out of either fingering wool or crochet cotton. Nearly any lacy knit or crochet pattern can be adapted to make a suitable and decorative exterior for the herbs. For those who do not knit or crochet, bobbin lace is another time-honored skill that makes beautiful fabric in which to put the liner-pouch full of herbs.

Thrift shops can be absolutely delightful treasure troves for finding useful materials for an heirloom feel without a handmade covering. Crocheted doilies can be wrapped around the lining bags to create wonderfully ornate pouches. Old lace curtains (preferably cotton ones) could be used like this as well. Resale shops are also great resources for finding additional supplies to be used for herbal pouches, such as ribbons, buttons, and beads. Using two coverings for the herbs—the liner and the decorative exterior—means that the outer layer of the pouch can be removed and cleaned, leaving the inner bag still intact.

Personalizing the sachet to the recipient is a great way to give a gift that is both useful and meaningful. The colors and patterns of the exterior can be chosen to reflect the person's tastes. Even the herbs and flowers in the pouch, through their traditional meanings, can send a message of love, support, or friendship.

Making herbal sachets is great fun as a group activity, and it may even become quite addictive. Everyone can bring some materials to share, and a collection of different sachets can be made for keeping and for giving to others. Perhaps seasonal sachets can be made at different times of the year, or the herbs can be themed for various occasions. Whether done in groups or working solitary, this is one of the old-fashioned crafts that is worthy of reviving and preserving.

Herbal References

Arrowsmith, Nancy. *Essential Herbal Wisdom*. Llewellyn, 2009.

Black, Penny. *The Book of Potpourri*. Simon & Schuster, 1989.

Lehner, Ernst and Johanna. *Folklore and Symbolism of Flowers, Plants and Trees*. Dover Publications, 2003.

Long, Jim. *Making Herbal Dream Pillows*. Storey Publishing, 1998.

Lace References

Dye, Gilian, and Adrienne Thunder. *Beginner's Guide to Bobbin Lace*. Search Press, 2008.

Hubert, Margaret. *Lacework for Adventurous Crocheters*. Creative Publishing International, 2013.

Weiss, Rita. *50 Fabulous Knitted Lace Stitches*. Leisure Arts, Inc., 2009.

Charlie Rainbow Wolf *is happiest when she is creating something, especially if it can be made from items that others have cast aside. Pottery, writing, knitting, and Tarot are her deepest interests, but she happily confesses that she's easily distracted because life offers so many wonderful things to explore. Charlie is the Dean of Faculty at the Grey School, where she teaches subjects in most of the sixteen departments. She is an advocate of organic gardening and cooking, and lives in the Midwest with her husband and special-needs Great Danes. Visit her at www.charlierainbow.com.*

Tiny Worlds: Designing and Creating Your Own Terrariums

⤜ By Deborah Castellano ⤛

My great-aunt's house was a place of wonders but also trials. My cousins and I liked to skitter around the basement, causing as much of a ruckus as my great-aunts and grandmother would permit. That is, until we started weaving around them in the second kitchen in the basement like sugar-crazed cats, thanks to the cookies or cake we were permitted for breakfast (we're Italian-American, in case you can't tell!). When we crossed the threshold from playful to annoying, we were unceremoniously thrown out into the backyard of Aunt Anna's house with the one toy we were allowed—a rubber ball so old that one of my cousins' mothers remembered playing with

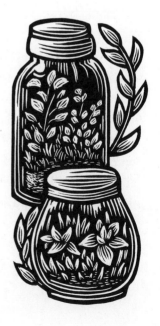

it as a child. We would dejectedly throw the ball around in the cold or the rain until we were allowed back inside. Then I would slink off to the front entryway, grandly called the "sunroom."

My aunt had a lot of plants, so it was fun to pretend that I lived in a jungle in the front room, but mostly, I was entranced by her terrariums—the pretty rainbow sand at the bottom, the spikiness of the cacti, and the saucy, tiny porcelain animals that lived in this sexy little desert. I could be lost in terrarium adventures for as long as I was permitted.

By the time I was a teenager, there was nothing cool about terrariums; they seemed hopelessly outdated and mid-century kitsch. Perhaps my teenage self would have been more enticed if I had known the true origins of the terrarium. The earliest recorded terrarium came from the Victorian era. Dr. Nathaniel Bagshaw Ward was a physician with a love of the great outdoors. After conducting a moth cocoon experiment where he sealed the cocoons inside a glass case, he decided to have a carpenter build him a glass and wood case that looked something like a mini-greenhouse so he could see how ferns would grow in that environment. He soon saw that his case was the perfect environment for his ferns to grow and thrive. These cases were eventually called Wardian cases and caught on with professional gardeners to transport their plants to faraway buyers. From there, Victorian city dwellers started using the cases to grow ferns and orchids. The Wardian case soon came in a variety of different styles and shapes and eventually became the template for modern terrariums, which are considered a type of vivarium (Latin for "place of life"). Lidded terrariums are great examples of what a closed ecosystem should look like, which make them perfect for amateur botanists of all ages.

Eventually, I found that I really enjoyed the detail that goes into terrarium making. I'm a crafter by trade, but I generally don't sell my terrariums; it's an art I make for myself. When I feel completely stressed out, concentrating on terrarium making really helps me feel calm and like I can control something, even if it's just a small glass jar. I find creating terrariums to be more imaginative than standard gardening. Even if you live in a dorm room or a studio apartment, you can create tiny indoor gardens to enjoy.

Figure out where you want to put your terrarium. The phrase "shade plant" can be deceptive. I thought that my moss would do fine in my dining room, which receives sunlight through my living room. This was a wrong assumption, as my dead moss can affirm. If you are putting your terrarium in a room without windows or a room that doesn't receive much sun regularly, your best bet would be to not include live plants.

The hardest aspect to learn, in my opinion, is scale. Generally speaking, make sure your plants or other "tall" objects are only half as tall as your container. So if your Mason jar is twelve inches tall, your plants or other tall objects should be six inches or smaller. Your miniature figurines should be smaller than three inches.

Clear glass containers are best to use for your terrarium so you can see everything inside it. Let your imagination go wild! Anything from apothecary jars to bell jars to Mason jars make good homes for terrariums.

Succulent plants such as baby toes, *Sedum burrito* (burro's tail), miniature aloe, and cactus plants do best in a fishbowl-style, lidless terrarium. Succulents need a lot of light and can be watered once a week. With the renewed popularity of terrariums, succulents are easy to find at your local garden center store or even your grocery store.

Mosses such as reindeer moss, sheet moss, pillow moss, and mood moss do best in lidded glass terrariums. Dried moss is great to use if your terrarium is in a place without sunlight, but live moss needs some sunlight. Live moss can be found in your own backyard or ordered online from a place like Etsy. Live moss won't directly root to your soil, but it does have tiny threads that will anchor to your soil. Live moss should be misted with water once a week.

The best kind of soil to use for your terrarium is a soil mix that is made specifically for container gardening. You can purchase this kind of mix at your local garden store. Colored or white sand can make a pretty decorative top layer for your succulent terrarium or as a contrast layer between the stone layer and soil layer in your moss terrarium.

Stones are crucial to provide your terrarium with proper drainage. You can get smooth stones from your local craft store. The stone layer always goes at the bottom of the terrarium. Remember to consider scale when selecting your stones. Tiny pebbles are perfect for smaller terrariums, and river stones for larger terrariums.

Figurines can be anything from tiny people to doll house furniture to tiny woodland creatures. If you're making a tiny terrarium, be sure to pick smaller-scale figurines. Figurines can be found at flea markets, model train stores, craft stores, garage sales, dollar stores, and vintage shops.

If sunlight is an issue in your living space, you can still make a terrarium. Consider using items such as dried moss, figurines, colored sand, tumbled stones, pinecones, and dried flowers.

For the Love of a Fawn: A Terrarium That Does Not Require Sunlight

Supplies:

- 1 ounce of tiny pebbles in the color of your choice
- 1 ounce of sand in the color of your choice
- One 8-ounce wide-mouth glass jar
- A small selection of dried moss and lichen
- A few tiny pinecones
- 1–2 tiny plastic deer figurines, 1 inch or smaller (I like to paint mine gold)

Pour the pebbles and then the sand into the glass jar. Arrange the moss, pinecones, and deer until you're happy with the way it looks, remembering to keep the top half of your jar empty so the scale will be correct. Keep the lid off this jar and display on a low space, such as a desk, window ledge, coffee table, or low bookcase.

Route 66: A Succulent Terrarium

Supplies:

- ¼ cup medium-size river stones
- 10-inch glass bubble bowl (a goldfish-style bowl)
- 4 succulent plants, 2-inch size (baby toes and sedum look good together)
- 2 cups cactus soil
- ½ cup white sand
- ¼ cup tiny black pebbles
- Toy car of your choice

Place the river stones at the bottom of the glass bubble bowl. Arrange the succulents as you desire. Add the soil. Add the sand on top of the soil in an even layer. Use the tiny black pebbles to shape a road from one side of the bowl to the other. Put the car on top of the pebbles. Place near a sunny window.

The Little Prince: An Aquatic Terrarium

Supplies:

¼ cup small seashells

1 small lidded apothecary jar

¼ cup white sand

2 small marimos (A marimo is a small aquatic moss ball that is found in Japan. Marimos represent enduring love, as they grow very slowly every year. They also bring good luck. They need at least some sunlight, and their water should be changed once a week. They can be purchased online.)

Distilled water

Place the seashells in the apothecary jar, then add the sand and marimos. Fill the jar with distilled water and put the lid on. Place it in a room that gets sunlight but keep out of direct sunlight.

Rabbit-Hearted: A Moss Terrarium

Supplies:

½ cup small pebbles

1 tall apothecary jar with lid

1 cup container garden soil

A variety of live moss (mood and cushion moss look
  very nice together)

A few small rabbit figurines

A few small crystal points (such as quartz, amethyst, etc.)

Put the pebbles at the bottom of the terrarium and add the soil.
Arrange your live moss in whatever fashion you like, then add
the rabbit figurines and crystal points. Put the lid on the terrarium and keep it on unless you're watering your moss. Make
sure to put your moss terrarium in a room that gets a decent
amount of direct sunlight.

Oh-So-Zen Sand Terrarium: A Terrarium That Does Not Require Sunlight

Supplies:

1 rectangular glass container with lid

1 cup natural sand

1 chopstick

Small pieces of driftwood

A few white stones

A small Buddha figurine

Lay the container on its side near to where you want to display
it. Pour in the sand and use a chopstick to arrange the sand.
Use the chopstick to place the driftwood, stones, and Buddha
wherever you like them best. Put the lid on and carefully place
the terrarium where you want it to be. A higher spot, like a
high shelf or bookcase, would be a good place for this particular terrarium.

Light and Airy Terrarium

Supplies:

¼ cup small white pebbles

1 hanging glass terrarium (can be bought at a craft shop)

¼ cup sand

Air plants, also known as *Tillandsia* (Air plants need to be misted with water a few times a week and need sunlight, despite what the name implies. They don't really need soil, however, and should be placed near a window. They can be bought online and at some specialty shops.)

Put the pebbles at the bottle of the glass terrarium container and then add the sand. After that, add the air plants. Hang near a window.

Bibliography

Geiger, Kat. *Terrariums Reimagined*. Ulysses Press, 2013.

Martin, Tovah. *The New Terrarium*. Martin & Clineff, 2009.

Wardell, Randy A. *Patterns for Terrariums and Planters*. Wardell Publications, 1987.

Wilson, Charles L. *The World of Terrariums*. Jonathan Davis Publishers, 1975.

Deborah Castellano *enjoys writing about earth-based topics, though she has been known to write romantic fiction as well. Her craft shop, La Sirene et Le Corbeau, specializes in handspun yarn and other goodies. She resides in New Jersey with her husband, Jow, and two cats. She has a terrible reality television habit she can't shake and likes St. Germain liqueur, record players, and typewriters. Visit her at www.deborahmcastellano.com.*

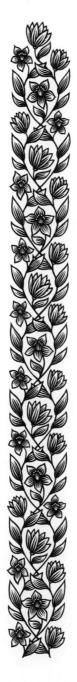

Herb History,
Myth, and Lore

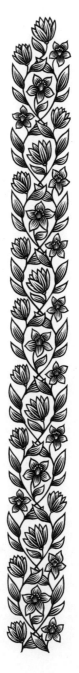

What the Old Wife Knew: Gardening Tips That Work

❧ By JD Hortwort ❧

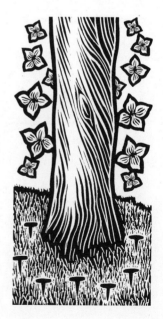

W e've all grown up with them—
the habits and recommendations that never seem to have much
of a basis in fact. We only have the
assurance from our elders that "this
always worked for my grandma (or
uncle or great-aunt or that old farmer
who lived on the dirt road)."

They are old wives' tales, which,
oddly, didn't always come from old
wives. They are the legend and lore
that fuel our gardening routines and
give us hope when modern solutions
seem to fail.

And let's face it—some of those
old wives were pretty smart old birds.
Some old wives' tales work. Many

don't. But the ones that fail are quickly forgotten or forgiven when some obscure tip from a wizened fellow gardener pans out.

My own mother did not have much of a green thumb. She didn't care for vegetable gardening, but she did love her flowers. As a perennial novice, anything that seemed to suggest success got put to the test in her woody landscape.

One item she coveted was a pink flowering dogwood. This was in the days before many of the reliable pink hybrids of *Cornus florida* that are available today. One or two could be seen in the local feed and seed store, but they were expensive, and for us, money was tight.

A great-aunt from down in the country told my mother that she could turn her white dogwoods pink if she drove iron nails into the ground around the dogwood roots. That was a cheap-enough fix for Mama. She scrounged rusty nails from every old board she could find. With hammer and nails in hand, we all took turns pounding the nails well into the ground around the dogwood outside her bedroom window.

Sure enough, in a couple of years Mama was rewarded with pink-tinged flowers on her white dogwood. The color wasn't pervasive. Only the veins of the bracts were affected. But from a distance, you could see a definite pink haze on one tree that stood out against the white dogwood flowers in the surrounding forest.

This was one time the old wife didn't let us down.

Soil Improvements

Mama's tip involved changing something in the soil. In this case, she added iron to the soil. Dogwoods are acid-loving and do not perform well in iron-deficient soil. We may have overloaded the tree with iron, and that showed up in the flowers.

The effect lasted only a couple of years, suggesting that the excess iron eventually leached out or was used up. Regardless, Mama was happy with the result.

Several old wives' tales involve making changes to the soil. When it comes to gardening, you've got to start at the bottom. The soil is the thing that will make or break your vegetable patch, flowerbed, or landscape.

Everyone has their own favorite old wives' tale for fueling success in the garden. Some of these are based on real science.

Take the tip that encourages gardeners to add eggshells or powdered milk to vegetable beds, especially tomato patches. Both are said to prevent blossom-end rot, which is the condition where a tomato looks beautiful near the stem and shoulders but the fruit has a sunken, black, decayed spot on the bottom or blossom side. This can happen to a lot of vegetables besides tomatoes, including peppers, squash, melons, and eggplant.

Blossom-end rot is caused by environmental factors, one of which is a heavy, poorly drained soil. If the plant is struggling to develop a strong root system, it can't deliver the proper nutrients to the fruit. Another factor is a lack of calcium—and this is where the lightbulb goes off! Eggshells and powdered milk have plenty of calcium. If you make sure plenty of calcium is available when the plant is set in the ground, then even a poorly developed root system should be able to access what it needs to make a tasty, healthy tomato.

This will only get you so far. No substitute exists for a well-prepared planting area. Add all the eggshells you want to a plant hole dug in heavy soil, but if the soil becomes saturated with too much rain, your tomatoes will likely still develop some problems with blossom-end rot. But adding these amendments to a good planting soil will increase your odds of success.

Epsom salt is another favorite of the old wife. Are your plants puny? Do they appear weak and wilted? Add a tablespoon of Epsom salt to the soil when planting, or water them with a solution of Epsom salt (one tablespoon to a gallon of water). That should fix the plants right up!

And it will—if the problem is a deficiency of magnesium. Epsom salt is magnesium sulfate. Plants need magnesium for strong cell-wall growth, seed germination, photosynthesis, and fruit production. Generally, soils have enough magnesium, and what they lack is made up for in the fertilizer we apply. So while Epsom salt can add magnesium to the soil, you usually don't need it. Testing the soil for an imbalance is better than applying Epsom salt willy-nilly. The reason is, while too much magnesium won't cause a direct problem, it can cause other troubles. Too much magnesium can interfere with the absorption of calcium, which leads us right back to that blossom-end-rot condition mentioned earlier.

In this case, the old wife needs to look for other solutions for her stunted plants.

What other soil additives does the old wife use?

Ashes from the Fireplace

Wood ash adds potassium to the soil. Grandma used to send us out to the garden in the winter to scatter cold wood ash from her stove. Use it in moderation, however. Potassium moves through the soil slowly. It generally only needs to be added every two to three years.

Coffee Grounds or Tea Leaves

Using these remnants in the garden isn't bad. It's kind of like compost. The small amount the average family has left over from the morning coffee or pitcher of tea won't hurt. It won't especially help any more than any other type of compost, but it won't hurt. The problem comes with adding coffee grounds or tea leaves to houseplants. Both end products are very acidic. You can quickly overload a house plant and end up with yellowing of foliage (chlorosis). Better to chuck these leftovers into the compost pile.

Sugar

The idea is that the sugar feeds the beneficial micro-organisms in the soil that help plants to thrive. Despite the testimony of some growers, adding sugar to plant water causes more problems than benefits. Sugar upsets the soil's pH balance. It can interfere with the plant's natural ability to make its own sugars and disrupt photosynthesis. Frankly, people are too hooked on sugar—we don't need to make addicts out of our plants.

Urine

Believe it or not, some gardeners like to add human urine to their compost pile and sometimes directly to the root zone of their plants. While it might sound gross, animal urine is already used to make fertilizer, because urine is a good source of nitrogen. The World Health Organization says the urine of a healthy person used in conjunction with compost should pose no health risk when the compost is properly handled—preferably with gloves and a long-handled pitchfork. The old wife or, in this case, the old farmer was on to something. But check with your local Cooperative Extension office about details and your local homeowners' association about restrictions.

Insect and Pest Control

Our old wife really comes into her own with recommendations about insect and pest control. One tale I've heard often is, put spearmint chewing gum in the run of a mole or vole. The critter is thought to eat the gum. The gum "gums up" the animal's digestive system and it dies—except moles are insectivores that don't eat plant material, much less chew gum. Voles are plant eaters, but there is no evidence that they are tempted by chewing gum either. So much for that old tale!

Moles and voles are a favorite target of the old wife. You may have heard that sticking pinwheel fans into the ground creates vibrations that scare away moles. Or perhaps you've heard of dropping castor bean seeds into vole runs. Neither of these "cures" works. Trying to flush the runs out with water doesn't either. A good hunting cat or energetic dog—these work. They also get you around a very interesting restriction. Some moles are considered endangered species, and it is illegal for you to trap or kill them. The rules say nothing about an attack dog.

Here are some other popular remedies:

Plant Companions

This is a lovely idea. Certain plants, when planted together, are supposed to act as guardians to each other. For example, broccoli grown near cucumbers is said to repel striped cucumber beetles. Onions are thought be to a good companion to carrots. Amaranth is thought to keep leaf miners away from bell pepper plants. Author Louise Riotte made a name for herself with her books on the topic, beginning with *Roses Love Garlic*. Since then, many organic-gardening websites have taken up the banner and offer a wealth of recommendations ready for you to test out.

Marigolds

This companion plant is legendary and deserves a special note. Planting marigolds is said to keep beetles off beans and cucumbers and nematodes away from all kinds of veggies. Not just any marigold will work, however. The old wife would use *Tagetes patula* (French marigold) or *Tagetes erecta* (African marigold). Some modern hybrids have lost the chemical signature that makes the marigold a good bug repellent. Pot marigold doesn't work either. It's not even in the *Tagetes* family. It is *Calendula officinalis*.

Homemade Insecticidal Sprays

Gardeners could fill a book with recipes for home insect sprays. One of the oldest taught to us by the old wife is made with lye soap. It is especially effective on soft-bodied insects, like aphids and mealy bugs. The fatty acids that make up lye soap break down the insect's exoskeleton. A quick recipe is to grate a bar of lye soap to get four tablespoons of flakes. Put these in a pint jar with two cups boiling water. Allow the soap to dissolve. Mix one to two tablespoons of this mixture with one quart of water to spray on plants. Just don't use it when temperatures are over 90 degrees Fahrenheit; don't use on tender young plants and don't use on fruit trees.

White Paint or Chalk

As a child, I remember seeing whole neighborhoods in which the tree trunks were painted white from the roots up to about chest high on an adult. I remember seeing an elderly neighbor lady diligently outlining her door frames and windowsills with white chalk. Both of these efforts were to keep bugs away, specifically ants in the old lady's case. White paint on tree trunks is a holdover from when farmers used to paint orchard trees with lime sulfur to kill insect eggs and scale insects. Over time, people forgot about the lime sulfur and seem to have assumed that any white paint would do. It works a little too well. Latex can suffocate plant cells along with the insects, damaging the tree. The white chalk is another matter. The thought is that the chalk might disrupt the scent trails that ants lay down. Another proposal is that on vertical surfaces, powdery chalk doesn't give ants the traction they need to climb. At best, this solution works only marginally and has to be reapplied regularly.

Planting by the Moon

No discussion of old wives' tales would be complete without mention of planting by the moon signs. My grandma swore by them. My father swore it was all bunk! We grew up calling it "planting by the signs." Now it's called "astro-gardening."

The belief is that the moon has an effect on plants as it goes through its 28-day cycle of waxing and waning. The effect is tempered by the zodiac signs through which the moon travels as it progresses through the sky.

The rules can be extensive. Plant above-ground crops under the waxing moon. Plant below-ground crops under the waning moon. Pull or cut weeds when the moon is in Leo. Plant fruit crops when the moon is in Pisces. Prune in the third or fourth quarter of the moon. The list goes on.

Science is largely silent on the issue. Some limited research exists on the impact of light on weed seed germination. Researchers found that fields tilled in the dark of the moon had less weed seed germination than fields tilled by the light of the moon. Limited studies seem to suggest that seeds of all sorts germinate better when planted under a waxing moon. But that is the extent of it.

It seems the old wife will have the last say on this one, for now.

There seems to be no end to the tales the old wife tells in the garden. Some are true, some are not. Watering midday won't scorch your plants, as she would tell you, but don't do it anyway. Too much water is lost to evaporation. Wait until the next morning. Coffee grounds won't keep slugs away from your hostas, but mulching the soil with sweetgum balls will. A bag of water hung outside your screen door won't keep the flies away, but a tall, narrow-neck bottle with a little apple cider inside will lure many flying insects to a watery grave.

I suppose we all contribute to the accumulation of old wives' tales as we age. The old wife probably never heard of using Listerine to repel mosquitoes (doesn't work) or Avon's Skin So Soft (this doesn't either, but Avon won't confirm or deny). But there is always an adventurous person out there ready to test the boundaries of common everyday products to give us the next generation of old wives' tales.

JD Hortwort *resides in North Carolina. She is an avid student of herbology and gardening. JD has written a weekly garden column* *for over twenty years. She is a professional, award-winning writer, journalist, and magazine editor and a frequent contributor to the Llewellyn annuals.*

For the Love of Violets

≫ By Charlie Rainbow Wolf ≪

Mark Twain once said, "Forgiveness is the fragrance that the violet sheds upon the heel that crushes it." We can learn even more what the author meant by this when we look into the gentle history and symbolism of this blossom. Violets have long been associated with compassion, love, and purity. There's much more to this humble flower than meets the eye, though.

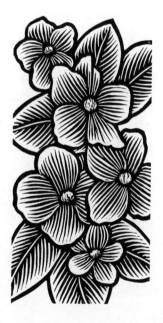

Folklore is peppered with information about violets; they have been included in songs, sonnets, and poems from Greek mythology onward. They are associated with Venus, the planet of beauty and love. A gift of violets from a lover is a very good omen, and to dream of violets indicates that marriage to a younger person is probable.

Violets belong to the Violaceae family, and there are both wild and cultivated types, although the cultivars are indeed off-spring of their wild relatives. The *Viola* genus has in excess of four hundred varieties, ranging in color, size, and scent. Violets will freely cross-pollinate, often making exact identification difficult. Wild violets do share most of the same habits and growing patterns, although domestic violets may be significantly more finicky. (Note: the African violet—*Saintpaulia*—is not a violet at all, it is only named so because of the appearance of the blooms, and should not be confused with other violets.)

For the most part, wild violets are perennial, blooming in the spring but occasionally in the autumn, too. Most varieties have waxy, heart-shaped leaves and a deep root system that can be hard to eradicate. Their normal growth is about five inches tall, although taller—and wider—varieties are not uncommon. The seedpods will split when ripe, dispersing the seeds to begin new plants. Wild violets prefer shaded areas, with moist and fertile soil. Many consider this humble flower to be a weed because of its tendency to invade lawns and wooded areas of the garden. Various types of helpful insects, such as bees and butterflies, are attracted to violets, and thus these flowers can be called a beneficial (companion) plant. Wild violets are not plagued by many problems, but, like their cultivated counterparts, they can be affected by mildew, mold, and fungus issues due to the damp areas in which they like to grow.

Wild violets bloom in white, yellow, pale mauve, right through to the deepest amethyst, and not just the purple petals that are usually associated with them. They all share the same qualities, but some shades are more common than others. Obviously, when using the flowers in crafts or culinary arts, the different colors are going to influence the outcome of the project.

While some people might consider the violet a nuisance, others are discovering just how delightfully versatile this humble flower can be. Long before pharmaceutical companies were producing pills and potions, the healing qualities of the violet were greatly valued. Hippocrates mentioned using violets as early as 466 BCE.[1] In his herbal, Nicholas Culpeper extols the virtues of the violet, saying that it eases pain, dissolves swelling, aids the liver, assists the lungs, and more.[2] Modern-day homoeopathists still have use for this gentle plant.

Violets are beneficial to the garden, even though they may not be appreciated there. If the violet is considered to be an opportunistic plant, then it is going to grow where it is most in harmony with its environment. There is a school of thought that these supposedly invasive plants can help to restore the natural balance of their environment. In his book *Invasive Plant Medicine*, Timothy Lee Scott says, "All colonizing plants offer medicine,"[3] so it would seem that the humble violet has much to offer us if we are willing to accept the gift.

Violet Recipes

In addition to being a pretty blossom and a sign that spring is arriving, the violet can also be used as a delightful kitchen ingredient. Recipes for violets are not often found in standard cookbooks. However, the diverse violet can add interest to many dishes—food or beverage, savory or sweet.

Violet Water

Violet water can be made similar to violet tea, by picking blossoms in the morning, before the sun has reached them. Place the flower heads in a glass jar, one that has a good lid. Make a tea by pouring boiling water onto the petals, and when it has cooled slightly, seal tightly. After about two days, open the jar and strain out the petals. The resulting water can then be used to add color and flavor to food. Try substituting it for rose water in Turkish delight for a delightfully different result.

Violet Syrup

Violet water can be used as the base for violet syrup. Put the water into a heavy-bottomed pan and add sugar (I use about two parts sugar to one part water, or about two cups sugar to every one cup violet water). Bring to a rolling boil, stirring constantly until all the sugar is dissolved. Cool completely, then refrigerate. This syrup is lovely on its own. As the base for a cordial, simply dilute it to taste and serve over ice. Add the juice of a lemon to the syrup and drizzle it over pancakes.

Violet Jam and Jelly

Jams and jellies do well with the violet treatment, too. I use violet water for the base, with a squirt of lemon juice added, and equal amounts of liquid to sugar. It has to boil for quite some time. Add liquid pectin, then very carefully pour the hot jelly into sterilized jars and seal using the hot-water-bath canning method.

Candied Violets

Candied violets are very easy to make. They are not a vegan treat, though, because they do use the beaten white of an egg.

Gather the flower heads early in the morning, when they are fresh and vibrant. Gently clean them by washing them in cool water, drying them on paper towels. Using a small artist's brush kept just for cooking purposes, gently coat both sides of the flower petals with an egg white that has been beaten with a drop of water to thin it. Dip each flower into extra-fine (castor) sugar, and ensure it is thoroughly coated—tweezers or tongs can be a real asset here, as the flower heads are small. Gently shake off the loose sugar, then dip into the sugar again. Place on a plate covered with wax or parchment paper, and dry in a slow oven (300–325°F) for about half an hour. When they are completely dry and cooled, store between layers of paper in an airtight container. They'll keep for up to a month but may lose their color as they age.

Violets are a lot more than just a spring flower or an annoying weed. When their true value is understood, they can be appreciated for their tenacity. What's more, the violet connects us with folklore, herbal medicines, culinary delights, and also a bit of self-examination. Next time you feel weedy, remember the violet and its assets, and know that you, too, are a well of hidden wonder, with assets and purpose just waiting for the right moment to bloom.

Notes

1. Nelson Coon, *The Complete Book of Violets* (London: AS Barnes & Company, 1977).

2. Nicholas Culpeper, *Culpeper's Herbal Remedies* (Wilshire Book Company, 1971).

3. Timothy L. Scott, *Invasive Plant Medicine* (Rochester, VT: Healing Arts Press, 2010).

Charlie Rainbow Wolf *is happiest when she is creating something, especially if it can be made from items that others have cast aside. Pottery, writing, knitting, and Tarot are her deepest interests, but she happily confesses that she's easily distracted, because life offers so many wonderful things to explore. Charlie is the Dean of Faculty at the Grey School, where she teaches subjects in most of the sixteen departments. She is an advocate of organic gardening and cooking, and lives in the Midwest with her husband and special-needs Great Danes. Visit her at www.charlierainbow.com.*

The Alliums

❧ By Suzanne Ress ❧

A long time ago, when I was little more than a toddler freely roaming the neighborhood on my side of the street, I discovered a marvelous clump of long green grass growing near a neighbor's porch door. When I tore off a tiny fistful, something magical happened: it smelled and tasted like onions! Thereafter, whenever I thought to do it, I would wander over and grab myself a little snack.

Then one day the neighbor telephoned my mother.

"I think Suzie has been eating my chives," she said.

My mother hung up the phone and, coming close to my face, asked if I had been eating Mrs. Wilson's

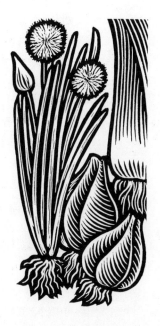

chives. Not knowing what chives were, I said no, but my mother knew the truth—she could smell them on my breath.

The most identifiable characteristic shared by species in the *Allium* genus is their oniony smell, which is not released unless the leaves or bulb are damaged, by cutting, trampling, tearing, or biting. Chives, garlic, leeks, onions, Welsh onions, garlic chives, scallions, shallots, and even some decorative alliums all contain cysteine sulfoxide, an amino-acid derivative that gives them their smell and taste.

Stinging nettles and poison ivy use a natural chemical reaction as their defense, triggered when the plant is damaged, or even just touched, to cause stinging and itching to the enemy (us). Alliums defend themselves with their pungent sulfuric smell, released when the plant feels threatened, to ward off attack. The onion (*Allium cepa*) has developed an extra line of defense: when cut, it releases syn-propanethial S-oxide, also known as "the lachrymator," which means "the tear maker." When this gas comes into contact with the water in your eyes, it forms sulfuric acid, which really stings!

Unfortunately for the alliums, especially *A. cepa*, human beings learned to love their taste and smell at least seven thousand years ago, and have been going whole hog ever since—onions are the second most produced and consumed vegetable in the world, after tomatoes.

Raw onions and garlic are used quite frequently in certain cuisines, particularly those from around the Mediterranean Sea area: Middle Eastern, Greek, Italian, Moroccan, etc. Their strong and persistent tastes are not to everyone's liking, nor can everyone easily digest raw onions and garlic. The more delicate flavors of alliums such as chives (*Allium schoenoprasum*), garlic chives (*Allium tuberosum*), scallions, and Welsh onions (both *Allium fistulosum*, though scallions are the young ones), which are almost always eaten raw, do not linger so long and are easier to digest.

Cooking garlic, onions, and leeks causes further chemical reactions that are very complex and not fully understood to this day. When cooked at higher temperatures, onions become caramelized. This is when their enzymes combine with their natural sugars and produce a lovely sweet taste almost like caramel candy.

Cooked onions play a part in virtually every type of cuisine. Open any cookbook to the section on long, slow pot cooking, be it American, French, Asian, Italian, or other, and inevitably the first listed ingredient is chopped onions.

The chemical properties in onions, garlic, and leeks work magically with carrots and celery when finely chopped in a *mirepoix* (the start of almost all stews and braised meat dishes) to transform the flavor of the meat and other ingredients into a whole that is greater than the sum of its parts. This is the creation of the delicious savory taste *umami*.

Many, even most, prepared and packaged savory food products and snacks contain some form of onion, garlic, or their flavoring, because the cooked allium taste is associated with the umami deliciousness principle.

On Sunday mornings, I compete in long-distance running competitions. So many times it has happened that I have found myself stuck behind a co-competitor who obviously ate a garlic-infused meal the night before that I now purposely avoid eating any garlic, cooked or raw, all day Saturday. Even taking a hot shower the morning after eating it does not get rid of the garlic smell if you sweat heavily. The fact that the scent of alliums, especially garlic, can remain intact for so many hours in a person's blood and sweat tells me that these sulfoxides are mighty potent indeed!

Ever since the beginning, even before human beings started cultivating them, allium plants have been highly valued for their healing properties and health benefits.

All of the alliums contain antibacterial and antifungal components, but naturally the strongest ones are the most potent. Onion and garlic extracts inhibit blood clotting and reduce cholesterol levels in people who have high-fat diets. They also reduce high blood pressure.

Many people add raw or dried garlic to their horses' feed in the spring to keep biting midges at bay. Although I've heard of people feeding garlic to dogs as a vermifuge, this may not be a good idea, as some sulfoxides cannot be digested by, and are toxic to, dogs. Cats should never be fed alliums of any kind.

Garlic contains allicin, a natural antibacterial that can be used in treating abrasions and superficial wounds. It is also effective against athlete's foot fungi and some of the viruses that cause colds and flu.

Garlic is also widely used in food preservation (think sausage, salami, pickles), together with salt and/or vinegar and/or hot peppers, for its bacteria-inhibiting ability as well as for flavor.

Allicin and the S-oxides are most potent in raw garlic and onions but are present in leeks, chives, scallions, and shallots, too. But be aware that microwave cooking destroys these natural chemicals!

With all of their health and flavor benefits, alliums truly pack a punch. But there is more: most edible alliums are high in calcium and vitamins A, C, and K, plus they have zero fat and are very low in calories.

Alliums, as a genus, are perennial bulbous plants with three important parts useful to humans: the bulb itself, the leaves, and the flower. As with amaryllis, which shares a family with the alliums (Amaryllidaceae), a solitary flower comes from each bulb. These are in the form of umbels, which usually form a globular shape on top of a long, straight stem.

The bulb is not a root, but a compressed stem covered with scaly leaves. In alliums such as garlic, onions, and shallots, it's the bulb we eat. The layers of leaves forming the bulb are particularly noticeable in the onion and scallion, but are even visible in garlic. The white part of a leek is its bulb, and in this allium, it's fascinatingly easy to see the layers of leaves that form the bulb. Even the tiny chive has a miniscule bulb.

Almost all alliums grow from bulbs, but there are a few exceptions. One of these is garlic chives (*Allium tuberosum*), which, as the name explains, has tuberous roots. I found this out the hard way, by planting a single clump of garlic chives in my herb garden one spring. I let its lovely white (and scented) flowers bloom, and then carelessly let them go to seed. Two years later, my herb garden contains a large section of invasive garlic chives, which are next to impossible to eradicate.

Garlic chives, like regular chives, are useful, though. I snip their tender leaves into little bits to strew over salads, fish, eggs, and summertime pasta dishes for a delicate garlic flavor.

There are many species of decorative alliums grown solely for their stately, dramatic flowers, which are globe-shaped and colorful. Probably the most well known of these is the happy-looking *Allium giganteum*, whose large round purple flower blooms atop a three-foot-tall stem in early summer. Several of these placed strategically in an herb garden are real attention grabbers. Other decorative alliums are *Allium sphaerocephalon*, with a striking two-toned burgundy and green cone-shaped flower; *Allium flavum*, which grows well in rock gardens and has drooping yellow umbels; and *Allium schubertii*, which has twelve-inch-wide globular pink umbels that look like fireworks. New *Allium* species are being developed by horticulturists all the time. Although the bulbs of decorative alliums can't be eaten, many of them still do give off the typical oniony or garlicky smell when damaged or rubbed. The flowers, highly attractive to butterflies and bees of all kinds, are usually unscented and can be successfully dried for lasting flower arrangements. And it's nice to know that if you happen to live near deer and rodent habitats, these animals will usually leave alliums alone.

The decorative alliums are hybrids—bred, inbred, and re-bred from their original state by human beings to favor large globular flowers or, in some cases, pretty drooping umbels, in a wide variety of colors. This inbreeding also tends to disfavor strong oniony odors. People started breeding flowering garden alliums in the late 1800s in Russia, and the passion soon spread to England and beyond. There are horticultural groups, or sections of groups, that specialize in alliums and the development of new ones. One of the newest cultivar creations is *Allium* 'Silver Spring' (2013). It has star-shaped, very pale green flowers with burgundy centers all over the four- to six-inch globes, and, surprisingly, smells like licorice candy.

From what we know, the most antique of all the alliums are *Allium sativum* (garlic), *Allium cepa* (onion), and *Allium porrum* (leeks), which were cultivated and used lavishly in Egypt, after having made their way there from Assyria, where systematic agriculture was born. Most likely, alliums originally came from Central Asia, as beloved wild plants. Even before alliums were cultivated, their wild relatives were favorite human foodstuff, far back into prehistoric times.

In ancient Egypt, onions, with their layers of leaves, symbolized eternity, and were buried along with important people, given as funeral offerings, offered to the gods, and served whole at banquets. Onions were placed in, on, or around various body parts of the dead. King Ramses IV, who died in 1150 BCE, was buried with onions placed in his eyes. It is believed that ancient Egyptians knew of onion's antiseptic properties.

In the Bible, Israelites speak of their preferred diet of onions, garlic, leeks, cucumbers, and melons.

Ancient Greek athletes fortified themselves for Olympic competition by eating copious amounts of raw garlic and onions. They also rubbed their muscles with cut onions and garlic, as an invigorating tonic. It's not hard to imagine what they must have smelled like!

The Romans loved garlic, onions, and leeks, as food and as medicine, believing them to cure problems of vision, insomnia, and the first signs of a cold.

In the Middle Ages, onions were used as a staple food, along with cabbage and beans, and as a medicine to cure headache and hair loss.

The Pilgrims brought onions with them on the Mayflower, but needn't have, for they found wild ones growing in New England. American Indians had already been using these wild onions for food, medicine, and dyes (golden yellows, oranges, and browns) for centuries.

The national emblem of Wales is the leek, because, during a battle against the Saxons, the Welsh patron saint David ordered his warriors to wear leeks on their helmets as identifying symbols. Shakespeare found this humorous, and often makes fun of the Welsh in his plays. There is a hilarious slapstick scene in *Henry V* (Act 5, Scene 1), on the battlefield, between Gower, Welshman Fluellen, and Pistol, which pokes fun at the leek in Fluellen's helmet (Fluellen suggests that Pistol eats it!). March 1 is Saint David's Day, celebrated by people of Welsh heritage all over the world by wearing and eating leeks.

There are known to be over 750 different species in the genus of *Allium*. Although alliums were originally placed in the Liliaceae family (along with lilies, asparagus, and crocii), in the more updated APG III classification system they have been placed in the Amaryllidaceae family.

Most alliums prefer sunny locations, a moderate climate, and average soil. They are fairly easy to grow. Bulbs should be planted in the fall, while chives and garlic chives should be set in, or divided, in spring. Alliums generally bloom in the summer, although a few ornamental species bloom in late spring or early fall. Leeks and scallions should be harvested before they are fully mature—before they flower, and when their leaves are still green and upright. The chives can be snipped at any time, and you can use the edible flowers, too, to decorate salads or cold soups. Onions and garlic are not ready for harvesting until their leaves begin to dry up and fall over. At that point, the bulbs can be dug up and used fresh, or left in a cool, dry place to dry for storage and later use.

Allium Recipes

Here are three of my favorite allium recipes.

Leek Salad for Saint Davy's Day

    8 leeks

    ⅓ cup olive oil

    2 tablespoons lemon juice

    1 clove garlic, very finely chopped

    1 teaspoon mustard

    1 handful fresh parsley, finely chopped

    Salt and pepper

Slice the white part of the trimmed and cleaned leeks into half-inch rounds. Drop them into boiling salted water for 8 minutes, then drain immediately and rinse in cold water. Put all the other ingredients into a jar with a lid. Close the lid and shake well, then pour this vinaigrette over the leeks and refrigerate. Serve on a bed of tender green lettuce leaves.

Roasted Whole Garlic

    Whole heads of garlic, 1 per person

    Olive oil

Heat the oven to 400°F. Trim the pointy ends from the garlic heads, and place each one on a square of aluminum foil. Drizzle a few drops of olive oil and a light sprinkle of salt on each head, then wrap them up tightly. Place all heads in a casserole dish. Put a little water on the bottom, cover the casserole, and bake for about 50 minutes. To eat, unwrap the foil and squeeze the softened garlic out of each clove onto fresh sourdough bread.

Onions Borettane

    1 ½ pounds pearl onions

    1 cup vegetable broth

1 tablespoon tomato paste

1 teaspoon brown sugar

1 tablespoon balsamic vinegar

3 tablespoons olive oil

Salt and pepper (optional)

Trim the onions, if necessary, then drop them into boiling water for 2 minutes. Drain, rinse in cold water, then put them into a large, heavy-bottomed pan. Add the vegetable broth, tomato paste, brown sugar, vinegar, and oil, and stir well. Heat on medium until the mixture comes to a boil. Turn down the heat and simmer 12 to 15 minutes, stirring regularly, until the liquid becomes quite dense. Season with salt and pepper, if desired. Stir and serve warm, as a side dish.

The alliums really have all bases covered: they are vegetables, herbs, and ornamental flowers, and they deserve to be given space in every garden.

And as for my childhood foraging passion, soon after my mother told me to stop eating the neighbor's chives, I discovered wild sorrel. But that's another story.

Suzanne Ress *recently published her first novel,* The Trial of Goody Gilbert. *When she is not writing, Suzanne enjoys herb gardening, beekeeping, creating mosaic artworks, silver and copper-smithing, horse riding, and long-distance running. She lives in the foothills of the Italian Alps with her husband, daughter, and many animals.*

The Romance of Rosemary

≫ By Laurel Reufner ≪

Beloved by cooks around the world, we use rosemary to flavor our soups, stews, chicken, fish, and roasts of all sorts. Skewers of its wood are sought after for grilling. Rosemary is probably one of the top five herbs in our homes today, but thousands of years before we brought it into our kitchens, it was revered for so many other uses and reasons.

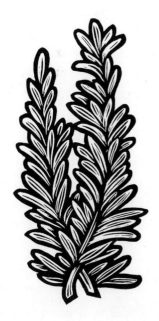

Egyptian tombs have been found to contain rosemary, including sprigs wrapped within the wrappings of some mummies. Greek students either wore chaplets of the herb or braided it into their hair to work as a study and memory aid. The Romans adorned their household gods, or Lares, with rosemary, believing that it promoted stability. The herb was also used in some temples as inexpensive and aromatic incense. (The French would later use it for the same purpose in their hospitals, and also hung branches about the wards.) On top of this, rosemary was valued in ancient gardens simply for its fragrance and beauty.

There is a lovely legend about how the Virgin Mary, while fleeing to Egypt, laid her blue cloak over a rosemary bush and rested in its shade. Thereafter, the flowers of the plant were blue out of appreciation for the honor she showed it. Furthermore, it is said that the rosemary will never grow taller than the age of Mary's son (the Christ) upon his death.

Moving on to the medieval period, rosemary's reputation as an aid to memory was drawn upon at both weddings and funerals, uses that lasted up until more modern times. Brides often carried sprigs of rosemary as part of their bridal bouquet, the branches of which would be gilded, or dipped in sweet or scented waters, as well as bound with colorful ribbons. Some brides wore rosemary woven into a chaplet for their hair.

In Elizabethan times, brides might be led to the church door by a pair of young lads who carried beribboned and gilded rosemary branches. The groom might wear a sprig of rosemary either upon his arm or his lapel. To further demonstrate rosemary's significance at such an important event, small sprigs of rosemary tied with even more ribbons were given to attendees to help them both celebrate and remember the day. In areas where rosemary couldn't be found, thanks to the high demand, broom would be substituted and used in a similar fashion.

Mourners en route to the cemetery would carry sprigs of rosemary, which were then tossed on the coffin before the grave was filled in. On some occasions even the corpse was decorated with rosemary. Even in some areas today, bits of rosemary are worn by mourners at a funeral, and it's a good choice for planting upon the gravesite of a loved one.

During this time period, rosemary was used in decorations of both banquet halls and churches. It was also popular for tossing during processions and parades, such as Queen Elizabeth's passage through London in 1558, during which she often stopped her carriage to receive one of the fragrant branches and an entreaty from someone along her route. Yet another example would be the arrival in London, in November 1640, of Masters Prynne and Burton, who had been imprisoned, among other penalties, for writing out against the British government at the time. Upon their release, thanks to a successful petition to Parliament by the wife of one of the other accused, they rode into the city with much celebration wearing wreaths of rosemary and bay.

Sprigs of rosemary, once again tied with ribbons and perhaps gilded, were also given at both Christmas and New Year's as tokens of friendly affection. A clove-studded orange often accompanied it.

And then there were the more extravagant claims of rosemary's uses. As the legend goes, in 1235, Queen Elizabeth of Hungary was suffering from paralysis. Her physician steeped one pound of rosemary in a gallon of wine (or perhaps brandy) and applied it to her limbs, thereby curing her. Hungary Water is now considered one of the very first alcohol-based fragrances, although it was still used medicinally, applied as a liniment, or drunk, for centuries. Later recipes came to include a variety of other herbs in addition to the rosemary, including rose, mint, sage, lemon, orange blossom, and marjoram. In the eighteenth century, rosemary's popularity was surpassed by eau de cologne, which also included rosemary essential oil.

Yet another miraculous medieval claim involving rosemary was the famous (infamous?) Four Thieves Vinegar. As the story goes, a group of thieves took to robbing graves around either Marseille or Versailles during the Black Death (in the fourteenth century). When they were eventually caught, people wondered how they had escaped contracting the plague during their grisly enterprises. In exchange for their lives (or perhaps for a merciful death, depending on the legend source), the grave robbers offered to reveal their secret for staying healthy and alive.

What's in Four Thieves Vinegar, you might ask? Well, according to a recipe said to have hung on the walls of Marseilles during the time of the plague, you will need three pints of strong white vinegar as well as two ounces each of angelica, rosemary, and horehound, a handful each of wormwood, meadowsweet, wild marjoram, and sage, plus three measures of camphor and fifty cloves. Allow it to steep for fifteen days and then strain and bottle.

Yet another recipe called for dried rosemary, sage flowers, lavender flowers, fresh rue, and camphor dissolved in an ethyl alcohol. Add some sliced garlic and bruised cloves, and place the whole lot in some wine vinegar. Let steep several days and then strain and bottle. To use either recipe, you simply rubbed it on hands, ears, and temples before encountering any plague sufferers. Of course, ridiculous discovery claims aside, Four Thieves did have some antiseptic properties that may have helped some people avoid catching the disease, especially since it was used on the hands. Four Thieves Vinegar still sees some use today, although mainly in the realm of spellcasting and magic.

Amazingly, rosemary could also help predict a person's romantic future. You will need one rosemary plant per potential lover, and it needs to be in its own pot. The plant that grows the fastest and strongest will be the person you marry. Actually, rosemary was so powerful that it was believed you could just use a sprig to tap the person you were interested in and they would fall for you. Also, a sprig of rosemary under your pillow at night was thought to ward off nightmares.

In the Victorian language of flowers, rosemary meant "remembrance"—at least in England. In France, it represented "reviving of one's spirit," which ties back in with its use as an incense and air purifier in hospitals.

Furthermore, rosemary grown in the garden was believed to protect a home from evil and the power of witchcraft. However, a thriving rosemary plant also meant that the woman of the house was the one to wear the pants. Some men may have sabotaged their wives' rosemary bushes so they couldn't be found wanting or thought to be weak.

In more modern times, rosemary sprigs are worn in Australia and New Zealand on ANZAC Day, April 25th, to commemorate both the brave efforts of their soldiers at the Battle of Gallipoli, during World War I, and to remember those who sacrificed their lives during the doomed battle for the Peninsula. Rosemary not only serves to remind Australians and New Zealanders of those lost, but it is also a reminder of where they died—along the Mediterranean Sea, where the shrub grows profusely.

And finally, rosemary was Napoleon Bonaparte's favorite scent.

There's rosemary, that's for remembrance; pray, love, remember.
—*Hamlet*, Scene IV, Act V

Bibliography

Brand, John. *Observations on the Popular Antiquities in Great Britain*. London: G. Bell, 1849.

Christian, Roy. *Old English Customs*. New York: Hastings House, 1966.

Lawson, James. "The Roman Garden." *Greece and Rome*. Vol. 19, No. 57 (Oct. 1950): 97–105.

Laurel Reufner *happily calls the gorgeous hills of Athens County, Ohio, home, where she lives with her husband and two daughters. She's been earth-centered for around twenty-five years now and enjoys writing about whatever shiny topics grab her attention, especially mythology and history. She is slowly working on editing her first book and hopes to have it finished by the time you read this. Keep up with her at her blog,* Laurel Reufner's Lair *(laurelreufner .blogspot.com) or like her Facebook page* Laurel Reufner.

The Hills of Frankincense

☙ By Linda Raedisch ❧

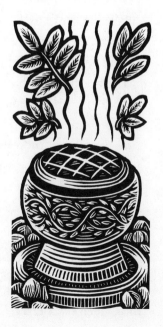

On one of the smaller panels of the fifth-century BCE Ludovisi triptych is a relief depicting a woman burning incense. Though she is sometimes described as a bride—perhaps because she is wearing a veil—more recent scholarship identifies her as an older woman. In ancient Greece (the triptych is in fact Greek, despite its Italian name), all women except slaves and prostitutes wore veils, and the Ludovisi lady wears hers pulled tight over her head and shoulders as she crouches before the *thymiaterion* to place a pinch of precious resin in the fire. A thymiaterion, from the ancient Greek *thymian*, "to smoke," is a censer raised on a pedestal so one might walk round it during the ritual offering of incense. This is not the sort of censer one would have at home, so the lady is probably participating in some public ritual, perhaps a festival in honor of Aphrodite. The Greeks adopted the burning of frankincense, myrrh, cinnamon, cassia, and other aromatics from the Persians, and by the fifth century BCE, incense had replaced the earlier practice of animal sacrifice.

Though her hand has been damaged, the woman is probably using her thumb, forefinger, and middle finger to pinch a bit of incense from the small receptacle, or *libanotris*, she holds in her left hand. In ancient Greece, this was the proper way to offer incense to the gods. *Libanos* is the ancient Greek word for frankincense. It comes from the South Arabian *libnay*, which also means frankincense and is derived from a Semitic root meaning "whiteness." This root also pops up in the modern Arabic *luban* and the English *olibanum*, both denoting the hardened resin of the frankincense tree. A libanotris could hold any kind of incense, so we cannot be sure what sort of resin she is about to offer to her deities. For the sake of this article, let us assume that it is in fact the whitish or "silver" resin of *Boswellia sacra*.

No one would rank *Boswellia sacra* among the world's one hundred or even one thousand most beautiful trees. It's barely a tree at all, but more like a shrub with aspirations. Its brave attempt at foliage consists of tiny, wrinkly leaves, and the flowers are nothing to speak of. All its worth lies beneath its gray bark. The frankincense tree does not grow in Greece or any other part of the Mediterranean. In fact, *Boswellia sacra*, the species that produces the finest grade of frankincense, grows only in the Dhofar Mountains of Oman and that part of Yemen that was once the land of Saba, or "Sheba." In English, the Queen of Sheba has no name, but in Arabic she has quite a few. One of them is Bal'amah, which may mean "incense." It comes from the same root as our word *balsam*. The Queen of Sheba's palace, along with her throne of ibex horns, has long since disappeared beneath the shifting dunes, but the resin that made the Sabaeans rich is still burned on portable horned censers throughout the South Arabian region.

The gates and towers of the oasis city of Ubar, too, have slipped beneath the sands. Ubar was an important stop along the incense road. Here, the straggling caravans stopped to water their camels and pay their tolls before setting off across the forbidding Empty Quarter with their cargoes. Along the old incense road, one can still find inscriptions in the Ubarites' South Arabian alphabet, whose letters, resembling lollipops, pitchforks, and stick-figure spacemen, must have been a joy to scratch into the rocks. Often, the merchants petitioned the gods to safeguard their cargoes of "incense," which, in Epigraphic South Arabian, was spelled Lollipop Bent-Stick Chicken-Foot Smoking-Chimney, but sometimes they simply wanted it to be known that they had been "here." In all the old tales, the Ubarites are referred to as the "People of 'Ad," and to this day the phrase "as old as 'Ad" expresses unimaginable antiquity. The descendants of the People of 'Ad, however, are alive and well, having retreated to the Dhofar Mountains and the source of all that ancient wealth. They are the Shahri, and they still speak the ancient, chirruping "language of birds," a Semitic tongue far older than Hebrew or classical Arabic that was once spoken within the walls of Ubar.

The Dhofar Mountains are a good place to raise a family, not just to harvest frankincense. It is the only part of Arabia that can support cattle, for the mountain meadows, watered by the monsoon rains, are lush with grass. It is a land of fig trees, foxes, and fresh mountain springs, each with its own guardian spirit who, in the old days, was appeased with offerings of food. On the dark side, witches are said to ride through the night on the backs of hyenas, disappearing into bat-haunted caves. And there are far too many snakes, one species of which, the carpet viper, can propel itself several feet into the air to deliver its lethal bite. In classical times, such "flying serpents" were believed to guard the sacred frankincense groves.

In this region of Southern Oman, the frankincense tree itself, which grows wild, is called *mughur*. In summer, the tree's bark is carefully scored and the sap allowed to slowly ooze to the surface. It must dry in the sun for a period of several days before the beads of hardened resin can be scraped off with a special knife. One of the best varieties of frankincense, they say, is the *hojary*, which is harvested near Hasik, a remote village lying in a crescent of mountains close by the sea. Back in the fifth century BCE, it could take as long as three months for the harvest of frankincense to reach the Mediterranean world from places like Hasik. By the time it arrived in the market stalls of Magna Graecia, this most highly desired of aromatics was worth its weight in gold.

Here at home in the twenty-first century, my little bag of hojary frankincense looks like a cross between rock candy and Turkish Delight. The scrotum-shaped lumps are yellowish rather than pure white and have a finish like frosted glass. They look more like something I might use to sweeten my tea rather than burn to supplicate the gods. I am not, you understand, an incense guru; I dabble in smudge sticks and stick incense and occasionally drop some loose cedar in a frying pan, but the burning of pure resins is new to me. It is with a sense of anticipation, then, that I open the bag for the first time, stick my nose inside, and inhale a clean, mild scent similar to turpentine.

I have carefully prepared my thymiaterion—a steep-sided pottery bowl lined with foil and placed over a tea warmer. I drop the first lump in the center of the charcoal tab and am soon rewarded as it turns the shiny yellow of chicken fat, bubbles around the edges, and commences lustily to smoke. As it burns, it releases a fragrance that is…nice. It reminds me of licorice (Good & Plenty, to be specific), with notes of eucalyptus and peppermint. It fails, however, to bowl me over, to transport me to the Dhofar Mountains, the Land of Sheba, or even to the campsite of the Magi with the Star of Bethlehem shining overhead. All in all, I am more impressed by the thickness and whiteness of the smoke than by the fragrance. Fearful of setting off the smoke alarm, my daughter—also a first-time frankincenser—and I decide to move the makeshift thymiaterion from the kitchen counter to the windowsill, where the smoke swirls joyfully out through the screen and ascends in twisting ribbons to the neighbors' windows and the gods. For about ten minutes, my little blue bowl is transformed into a cauldron of roiling smoke.

As my daughter and I stand, semi-entranced, before the window, we spot a young friend riding his bicycle in the apartment house parking lot. I would like to say that he is instantly drawn to the heady scents and billowing smoke of *Boswellia sacra*, but this is not the case.

"Can you see the smoke?" we call out to him. "Can you smell it?"

Our cyclist friend brakes just under the window and wrinkles his nose. "Smells kinda bad."

"It's frankincense," I explain. "You know, like 'gold, frankincense, and myrrh'? In ancient times it was worth its weight in gold."

"Did you have to pay a lot for it?" he asks.

I hold up my now-a-little-less-than-one-ounce of frankincense in its cellophane bag. "No, I didn't. I got all this for only $6.50, plus shipping and handling. And it came all the way from Oman. Ancient people just couldn't get enough of this stuff."

"Shame we don't have a time machine," he remarks, pedaling off again. By this time, my daughter has left the apartment to join him on her scooter.

But I am not finished. Frankincense was and still is used by the peoples of the Dhofar Mountains as a toothpaste, tooth filling, and chewing gum. Tooth filling and chewing gum would seem to me to be mutually exclusive properties, but the lesson is that frankincense is edible. In the classical world, it was most famously used to perfume the corpse as it burned on the funeral pyre, but the living also consumed it to cure all sorts of ailments. I select one of the smaller lumps from the bag, break off a tiny piece from the bulbous end, and bite down tentatively. No, it cannot be chewed like gum. The fragments make a nice home for themselves among my molars, where they slowly, very slowly, dissolve. (I suppose one could use it as a filling just until one could get to Ubar or the next large oasis and ask the local blacksmith to pull the offending tooth.) I have a sensation of menthol drifting up and out my nose, but as for taste...nothing. Maybe I'm missing something. I hurry outside and proffer tiny fragments to the kids. They're game—it really *does* look like candy—but since the cyclist is not my own child, I assure him, "They eat it in Oman. It's tree sap, just like maple syrup."

Unfortunately, they can't taste anything either, and my daughter soon spits hers in the arbor vitae. Well, actually, she places it, sticky and white, in the palm of my hand and I drop it in the arbor vitae. The cyclist sticks it out and eventually goes home with exotically freshened breath (another native use for frankincense), though I would be surprised if anyone notices.

Meanwhile, the resin in my pottery bowl has burned itself out, leaving behind a soft, fine white ash. Though you could hardly call my efforts a festival, I, like the veiled lady on the Ludovisi throne, have succeeded in making at least a semi-public offering of frankincense. I have also done my part to perpetuate the long-distance frankincense trade: though there were no camels, oases, or agoras involved, I *did* pay for shipping and handling. Since the days of Ubar, the worldwide demand for the resin of *Boswellia sacra* has fallen sharply, to say the least. Nowadays, most of the frankincense harvested by the Shahri and other tribes is for their own daily use, and many trees are no longer tapped at all. So, in ordering my little parcel from the Dhofar Governorate and burning the contents on a windowsill far from the hills of frankincense, I am helping to keep alive a tradition that is older than 'Ad.

Bibliography

Clapp, Nicholas. *The Road to Ubar: Finding the Atlantis of the Sands.* Boston: Houghton Mifflin, 1998.

———. *Sheba: Through the Desert in Search of the Legendary Queen.* New York: Houghton Mifflin Company, 2001.

Groom, Nigel. *Frankincense and Myrrh: A Study of the Arabian Incense Trade.* London and Beirut, Lebanon: Longman Group and Librairie du Liban, 1981.

Lawton, John. "Oman: Frankincense," *Saudi Aramco World* (May/June 1983), pp. 26–27.

"The Ludivisi Throne: A Description," www.collective.co.uk /thrones/htm/ludo.htm.

Mackintosh-Smith, Tim. "Scents of Place: Frankincense in Oman," *Saudi Aramco World* (May/June 2000), pp. 16–23.

Thomas, Bertram. *Arabia Felix: Across the Empty Quarter of Arabia*. New York: Charles Scribner's Sons, 1932.

Linda Raedisch's *most recent book for Llewellyn is* The Old Magic of Christmas: Yuletide Traditions for the Darkest Days of the Year. *She now incorporates frankincense in her own Yuletide traditions and aspires to become an incense guru. As an artist and author, Linda also finds much of her inspiration in the history of language and writing, preferring those alphabets that are undeciphered, lost, or simply forgotten. She lives in northern New Jersey.*

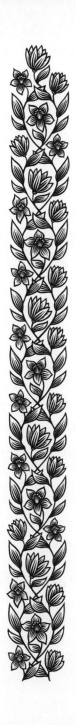

Moon Signs,
Phases, and
Tables

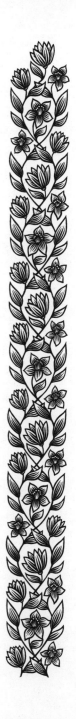

The Quarters and Signs of the Moon

Everyone has seen the moon wax and wane through a period of approximately 29½ days. This circuit from new moon to full moon and back again is called the lunation cycle. The cycle is divided into parts called quarters or phases. There are several methods by which this can be done, and the system used in the *Herbal Almanac* may not correspond to those used in other almanacs.

The Quarters

First Quarter

The first quarter begins at the new moon, when the sun and moon are in the same place, or conjunct. (This means the sun and moon are in the same degree of the same sign.) The moon is not visible at first, since it rises at the same time as the sun. The new moon is the time of new beginnings of projects that favor growth, externalization of activities, and the growth of ideas. The first quarter is the time of germination, emergence, beginnings, and outwardly directed activity.

Second Quarter

The second quarter begins halfway between the new moon and the full moon, when the sun and moon are at a right angle, or a 90° square, to each other. This half moon rises around noon and sets around midnight, so it can be seen in the western sky during the first half of the night. The second quarter is the time of growth and articulation of things that already exist.

Third Quarter

The third quarter begins at the full moon, when the sun and moon are opposite one another and the full light of the sun can shine on the full sphere of the moon. The round moon can be seen rising in the east at sunset, then rising a little later each evening. The full moon stands for illumination, fulfillment, culmination, completion, drawing inward, unrest, emotional expressions, and hasty actions leading to failure. The third quarter is a time of maturity, fruition, and the assumption of the full form of expression.

Fourth Quarter

The fourth quarter begins about halfway between the full moon and the new moon, when the sun and moon are again at a right angle, or a 90° square, to each other. This decreasing moon rises at midnight and can be seen in the east during the last half of the night, reaching the overhead position just about as the sun rises. The fourth quarter is a time of disintegration and drawing back for reorganization and reflection.

The Signs

Moon in Aries

Moon in Aries is good for starting things and initiating change, but actions may lack staying power. Activities requiring assertiveness and courage are favored. Things occur rapidly but also quickly pass.

Moon in Taurus

Things begun when the moon is in Taurus last the longest and tend to increase in value. This is a good time for any activity that requires patience, practicality, and perseverance. Things begun now also tend to become habitual and hard to alter.

Moon in Gemini

Moon in Gemini is a good time to exchange ideas, meet with people, or be in situations that require versatility and quick thinking. Things begun now are easily changed by outside influences.

Moon in Cancer

Moon in Cancer is a good time to grow things. It stimulates emotional rapport between people and is a good time to build personal friendships, though people may be more emotional and moody than usual.

Moon in Leo

Moon in Leo is a good time for public appearances, showmanship, being seen, entertaining, drama, recreation, and happy pursuits. People may be overly concerned with praise and subject to flattery.

Moon in Virgo

Moon in Virgo is good for any task that requires close attention to detail and careful analysis of information. There is a focus on health, hygiene, and daily schedules. Watch for a tendency to overdo and overwork.

Moon in Libra

Moon in Libra is a good time to form partnerships of any kind and to negotiate. It discourages spontaneous initiative, so working with a partner is essential. Artistic work and teamwork are highlighted.

Moon in Scorpio

Moon in Scorpio increases awareness of psychic power and favors any activity that requires intensity and focus. This is a good time to conduct research and to end connections thoroughly. There is a tendency to manipulate.

Moon in Sagittarius

Moon in Sagittarius is good for any activity that requires honesty, candor, imagination, and confidence in the flow of life. This is a good time to tackle things that need improvement, but watch out for a tendency to proselytize.

Moon in Capricorn

Moon in Capricorn increases awareness of the need for structure, discipline, and patience. This is a good time to set goals and plan for the future. Those in authority may be insensitive at this time.

Moon in Aquarius

Moon in Aquarius favors activities that are unique and individualistic and that concern society as a whole. This is a good time to pursue humanitarian efforts and to identify improvements that can be made. People may be more intellectual than emotional under this influence.

Moon in Pisces

Moon in Pisces is a good time for any kind of introspective, philanthropic, meditative, psychic, or artistic work. At this time personal boundaries may be blurred, and people may be prone to seeing what they want to see rather than what is really there.

January Moon Table

Date	Sign	Element	Nature	Phase
1 Thu 12:09 pm	Gemini	Air	Barren	2nd
2 Fri	Gemini	Air	Barren	2nd
3 Sat 8:08 pm	Cancer	Water	Fruitful	2nd
4 Sun	Cancer	Water	Fruitful	Full 11:53 pm
5 Mon	Cancer	Water	Fruitful	3rd
6 Tue 6:03 am	Leo	Fire	Barren	3rd
7 Wed	Leo	Fire	Barren	3rd
8 Thu 5:58 pm	Virgo	Earth	Barren	3rd
9 Fri	Virgo	Earth	Barren	3rd
10 Sat	Virgo	Earth	Barren	3rd
11 Sun 6:57 am	Libra	Air	Semi-fruitful	3rd
12 Mon	Libra	Air	Semi-sfruitful	3rd
13 Tue 6:44 pm	Scorpio	Water	Fruitful	4th 4:46 am
14 Wed	Scorpio	Water	Fruitful	4th
15 Thu	Scorpio	Water	Fruitful	4th
16 Fri 3:01 am	Sagittarius	Fire	Barren	4th
17 Sat	Sagittarius	Fire	Barren	4th
18 Sun 7:04 am	Capricorn	Earth	Semi-fruitful	4th
19 Mon	Capricorn	Earth	Semi-fruitful	4th
20 Tue 7:59 am	Aquarius	Air	Barren	New 8:14 am
21 Wed	Aquarius	Air	Barren	1st
22 Thu 7:48 am	Pisces	Water	Fruitful	1st
23 Fri	Pisces	Water	Fruitful	1st
24 Sat 8:31 am	Aries	Fire	Barren	1st
25 Sun	Aries	Fire	Barren	1st
26 Mon 11:37 am	Taurus	Earth	Semi-fruitful	2nd 11:48 pm
27 Tue	Taurus	Earth	Semi-fruitful	2nd
28 Wed 5:36 pm	Gemini	Air	Barren	2nd
29 Thu	Gemini	Air	Barren	2nd
30 Fri	Gemini	Air	Barren	2nd
31 Sat 2:09 am	Cancer	Water	Fruitful	2nd

February Moon Table

Date	Sign	Element	Nature	Phase
1 Sun	Cancer	Water	Fruitful	2nd
2 Mon 12:41 pm	Leo	Fire	Barren	2nd
3 Tue	Leo	Fire	Barren	Full 6:09 pm
4 Wed	Leo	Fire	Barren	3rd
5 Thu 12:46 am	Virgo	Earth	Barren	3rd
6 Fri	Virgo	Earth	Barren	3rd
7 Sat 1:44 pm	Libra	Air	Semi-fruitful	3rd
8 Sun	Libra	Air	Semi-fruitful	3rd
9 Mon	Libra	Air	Semi-fruitful	3rd
10 Tue 2:05 am	Scorpio	Water	Fruitful	3rd
11 Wed	Scorpio	Water	Fruitful	4th 10:50 pm
12 Thu 11:46 am	Sagittarius	Fire	Barren	4th
13 Fri	Sagittarius	Fire	Barren	4th
14 Sat 5:24 pm	Capricorn	Earth	Semi-fruitful	4th
15 Sun	Capricorn	Earth	Semi-fruitful	4th
16 Mon 7:13 pm	Aquarius	Air	Barren	4th
17 Tue	Aquarius	Air	Barren	4th
18 Wed 6:47 pm	Pisces	Water	Fruitful	New 6:47 pm
19 Thu	Pisces	Water	Fruitful	1st
20 Fri 6:13 pm	Aries	Fire	Barren	1st
21 Sat	Aries	Fire	Barren	1st
22 Sun 7:28 pm	Taurus	Earth	Semi-fruitful	1st
23 Mon	Taurus	Earth	Semi-fruitful	1st
24 Tue 11:54 pm	Gemini	Air	Barren	1st
25 Wed	Gemini	Air	Barren	2nd 12:14 pm
26 Thu	Gemini	Air	Barren	2nd
27 Fri 7:50 am	Cancer	Water	Fruitful	2nd
28 Sat	Cancer	Water	Fruitful	2nd

Times are in Eastern Time.

March Moon Table

Date	Sign	Element	Nature	Phase
1 Sun 6:34 pm	Leo	Fire	Barren	2nd
2 Mon	Leo	Fire	Barren	2nd
3 Tue	Leo	Fire	Barren	2nd
4 Wed 6:58 am	Virgo	Earth	Barren	2nd
5 Thu	Virgo	Earth	Barren	Full 1:05 pm
6 Fri 7:52 pm	Libra	Air	Semi-fruitful	3rd
7 Sat	Libra	Air	Semi-fruitful	3rd
8 Sun	Libra	Air	Semi-fruitful	3rd
9 Mon 9:10 am	Scorpio	Water	Fruitful	3rd
10 Tue	Scorpio	Water	Fruitful	3rd
11 Wed 7:30 pm	Sagittarius	Fire	Barren	3rd
12 Thu	Sagittarius	Fire	Barren	3rd
13 Fri	Sagittarius	Fire	Barren	4th 1:48 pm
14 Sat 2:40 am	Capricorn	Earth	Semi-fruitful	4th
15 Sun	Capricorn	Earth	Semi-fruitful	4th
16 Mon 6:14 am	Aquarius	Air	Barren	4th
17 Tue	Aquarius	Air	Barren	4th
18 Wed 6:58 am	Pisces	Water	Fruitful	4th
19 Thu	Pisces	Water	Fruitful	4th
20 Fri 6:28 am	Aries	Fire	Barren	New 5:36 am
21 Sat	Aries	Fire	Barren	1st
22 Sun 6:40 am	Taurus	Earth	Semi-fruitful	1st
23 Mon	Taurus	Earth	Semi-fruitful	1st
24 Tue 9:23 am	Gemini	Air	Barren	1st
25 Wed	Gemini	Air	Barren	1st
26 Thu 3:45 pm	Cancer	Water	Fruitful	1st
27 Fri	Cancer	Water	Fruitful	2nd 3:43 am
28 Sat	Cancer	Water	Fruitful	2nd
29 Sun 1:48 am	Leo	Fire	Barren	2nd
30 Mon	Leo	Fire	Barren	2nd
31 Tue 2:12 pm	Virgo	Earth	Barren	2nd

April Moon Table

Date	Sign	Element	Nature	Phase
1 Wed	Virgo	Earth	Barren	2nd
2 Thu	Virgo	Earth	Barren	2nd
3 Fri 3:07 am	Libra	Air	Semi-fruitful	2nd
4 Sat	Libra	Air	Semi-fruitful	Full 8:06 am
5 Sun 3:04 pm	Scorpio	Water	Fruitful	3rd
6 Mon	Scorpio	Water	Fruitful	3rd
7 Tue	Scorpio	Water	Fruitful	3rd
8 Wed 1:08 am	Sagittarius	Fire	Barren	3rd
9 Thu	Sagittarius	Fire	Barren	3rd
10 Fri 8:47 am	Capricorn	Earth	Semi-fruitful	3rd
11 Sat	Capricorn	Earth	Semi-fruitful	4th 11:44 pm
12 Sun 1:44 pm	Aquarius	Air	Barren	4th
13 Mon	Aquarius	Air	Barren	4th
14 Tue 4:12 pm	Pisces	Water	Fruitful	4th
15 Wed	Pisces	Water	Fruitful	4th
16 Thu 5:00 pm	Aries	Fire	Barren	4th
17 Fri	Aries	Fire	Barren	4th
18 Sat 5:31 pm	Taurus	Earth	Semi-fruitful	New 2:57 pm
19 Sun	Taurus	Earth	Semi-fruitful	1st
20 Mon 7:28 pm	Gemini	Air	Barren	1st
21 Tue	Gemini	Air	Barren	1st
22 Wed	Gemini	Air	Barren	1st
23 Thu 12:25 am	Cancer	Water	Fruitful	1st
24 Fri	Cancer	Water	Fruitful	1st
25 Sat 9:13 am	Leo	Fire	Barren	2nd 7:55 pm
26 Sun	Leo	Fire	Barren	2nd
27 Mon 9:07 pm	Virgo	Earth	Barren	2nd
28 Tue	Virgo	Earth	Barren	2nd
29 Wed	Virgo	Earth	Barren	2nd
30 Thu 10:03 am	Libra	Air	Semi-fruitful	2nd

Times are in Eastern Time.

May Moon Table

Date	Sign	Element	Nature	Phase
1 Fri	Libra	Air	Semi-fruitful	2nd
2 Sat 9:47 pm	Scorpio	Water	Fruitful	2nd
3 Sun	Scorpio	Water	Fruitful	Full 11:42 pm
4 Mon	Scorpio	Water	Fruitful	3rd
5 Tue 7:13 am	Sagittarius	Fire	Barren	3rd
6 Wed	Sagittarius	Fire	Barren	3rd
7 Thu 2:16 pm	Capricorn	Earth	Semi-fruitful	3rd
8 Fri	Capricorn	Earth	Semi-fruitful	3rd
9 Sat 7:22 pm	Aquarius	Air	Barren	3rd
10 Sun	Aquarius	Air	Barren	3rd
11 Mon 10:53 pm	Pisces	Water	Fruitful	4th 6:36 am
12 Tue	Pisces	Water	Fruitful	4th
13 Wed	Pisces	Water	Fruitful	4th
14 Thu 1:13 am	Aries	Fire	Barren	4th
15 Fri	Aries	Fire	Barren	4th
16 Sat 3:02 am	Taurus	Earth	Semi-fruitful	4th
17 Sun	Taurus	Earth	Semi-fruitful	4th
18 Mon 5:27 am	Gemini	Air	Barren	New 12:13 am
19 Tue	Gemini	Air	Barren	1st
20 Wed 9:56 am	Cancer	Water	Fruitful	1st
21 Thu	Cancer	Water	Fruitful	1st
22 Fri 5:42 pm	Leo	Fire	Barren	1st
23 Sat	Leo	Fire	Barren	1st
24 Sun	Leo	Fire	Barren	1st
25 Mon 4:52 am	Virgo	Earth	Barren	2nd 1:19 pm
26 Tue	Virgo	Earth	Barren	2nd
27 Wed 5:42 pm	Libra	Air	Semi-fruitful	2nd
28 Thu	Libra	Air	Semi-fruitful	2nd
29 Fri	Libra	Air	Semi-fruitful	2nd
30 Sat 5:34 am	Scorpio	Water	Fruitful	2nd
31 Sun	Scorpio	Water	Fruitful	2nd

June Moon Table

Date	Sign	Element	Nature	Phase
1 Mon 2:39 pm	Sagittarius	Fire	Barren	2nd
2 Tue	Sagittarius	Fire	Barren	Full 12:19 pm
3 Wed 8:50 pm	Capricorn	Earth	Semi-fruitful	3rd
4 Thu	Capricorn	Earth	Semi-fruitful	3rd
5 Fri	Capricorn	Earth	Semi-fruitful	3rd
6 Sat 1:02 am	Aquarius	Air	Barren	3rd
7 Sun	Aquarius	Air	Barren	3rd
8 Mon 4:16 am	Pisces	Water	Fruitful	3rd
9 Tue	Pisces	Water	Fruitful	4th 11:42 am
10 Wed 7:14 am	Aries	Fire	Barren	4th
11 Thu	Aries	Fire	Barren	4th
12 Fri 10:16 am	Taurus	Earth	Semi-fruitful	4th
13 Sat	Taurus	Earth	Semi-fruitful	4th
14 Sun 1:51 pm	Gemini	Air	Barren	4th
15 Mon	Gemini	Air	Barren	4th
16 Tue 6:51 pm	Cancer	Water	Fruitful	New 10:05 am
17 Wed	Cancer	Water	Fruitful	1st
18 Thu	Cancer	Water	Fruitful	1st
19 Fri 2:23 am	Leo	Fire	Barren	1st
20 Sat	Leo	Fire	Barren	1st
21 Sun 12:59 pm	Virgo	Earth	Barren	1st
22 Mon	Virgo	Earth	Barren	1st
23 Tue	Virgo	Earth	Barren	1st
24 Wed 1:41 am	Libra	Air	Semi-fruitful	2nd 7:03 am
25 Thu	Libra	Air	Semi-fruitful	2nd
26 Fri 1:57 pm	Scorpio	Water	Fruitful	2nd
27 Sat	Scorpio	Water	Fruitful	2nd
28 Sun 11:21 pm	Sagittarius	Fire	Barren	2nd
29 Mon	Sagittarius	Fire	Barren	2nd
30 Tue	Sagittarius	Fire	Barren	2nd

Times are in Eastern Time.

July Moon Table

Date	Sign	Element	Nature	Phase
1 Wed 5:11 am	Capricorn	Earth	Semi-fruitful	Full 10:20 pm
2 Thu	Capricorn	Earth	Semi-fruitful	3rd
3 Fri 8:21 am	Aquarius	Air	Barren	3rd
4 Sat	Aquarius	Air	Barren	3rd
5 Sun 10:23 am	Pisces	Water	Fruitful	3rd
6 Mon	Pisces	Water	Fruitful	3rd
7 Tue 12:38 pm	Aries	Fire	Barren	3rd
8 Wed	Aries	Fire	Barren	4th 4:24 pm
9 Thu 3:49 pm	Taurus	Earth	Semi-fruitful	4th
10 Fri	Taurus	Earth	Semi-fruitful	4th
11 Sat 8:16 pm	Gemini	Air	Barren	4th
12 Sun	Gemini	Air	Barren	4th
13 Mon	Gemini	Air	Barren	4th
14 Tue 2:14 am	Cancer	Water	Fruitful	4th
15 Wed	Cancer	Water	Fruitful	New 9:24 pm
16 Thu 10:15 am	Leo	Fire	Barren	1st
17 Fri	Leo	Fire	Barren	1st
18 Sat 8:47 pm	Virgo	Earth	Barren	1st
19 Sun	Virgo	Earth	Barren	1st
20 Mon	Virgo	Earth	Barren	1st
21 Tue 9:23 am	Libra	Air	Semi-fruitful	1st
22 Wed	Libra	Air	Semi-fruitful	1st
23 Thu 10:07 pm	Scorpio	Water	Fruitful	1st
24 Fri	Scorpio	Water	Fruitful	2nd 12:04 am
25 Sat	Scorpio	Water	Fruitful	2nd
26 Sun 8:24 am	Sagittarius	Fire	Barren	2nd
27 Mon	Sagittarius	Fire	Barren	2nd
28 Tue 2:47 pm	Capricorn	Earth	Semi-fruitful	2nd
29 Wed	Capricorn	Earth	Semi-fruitful	2nd
30 Thu 5:40 pm	Aquarius	Air	Barren	2nd
31 Fri	Aquarius	Air	Barren	Full 6:43 am

August Moon Table

Date	Sign	Element	Nature	Phase
1 Sat 6:36 pm	Pisces	Water	Fruitful	3rd
2 Sun	Pisces	Water	Fruitful	3rd
3 Mon 7:24 pm	Aries	Fire	Barren	3rd
4 Tue	Aries	Fire	Barren	3rd
5 Wed 9:29 pm	Taurus	Earth	Semi-fruitful	3rd
6 Thu	Taurus	Earth	Semi-fruitful	4th 10:03 pm
7 Fri	Taurus	Earth	Semi-fruitful	4th
8 Sat 1:40 am	Gemini	Air	Barren	4th
9 Sun	Gemini	Air	Barren	4th
10 Mon 8:08 am	Cancer	Water	Fruitful	4th
11 Tue	Cancer	Water	Fruitful	4th
12 Wed 4:52 pm	Leo	Fire	Barren	4th
13 Thu	Leo	Fire	Barren	4th
14 Fri	Leo	Fire	Barren	New 10:53 am
15 Sat 3:46 am	Virgo	Earth	Barren	1st
16 Sun	Virgo	Earth	Barren	1st
17 Mon 4:23 pm	Libra	Air	Semi-fruitful	1st
18 Tue	Libra	Air	Semi-fruitful	1st
19 Wed	Libra	Air	Semi-fruitful	1st
20 Thu 5:24 am	Scorpio	Water	Fruitful	1st
21 Fri	Scorpio	Water	Fruitful	1st
22 Sat 4:41 pm	Sagittarius	Fire	Barren	2nd 3:31 pm
23 Sun	Sagittarius	Fire	Barren	2nd
24 Mon	Sagittarius	Fire	Barren	2nd
25 Tue 12:22 am	Capricorn	Earth	Semi-fruitful	2nd
26 Wed	Capricorn	Earth	Semi-fruitful	2nd
27 Thu 4:03 am	Aquarius	Air	Barren	2nd
28 Fri	Aquarius	Air	Barren	2nd
29 Sat 4:51 am	Pisces	Water	Fruitful	Full 2:35 pm
30 Sun	Pisces	Water	Fruitful	3rd
31 Mon 4:33 am	Aries	Fire	Barren	3rd

Times are in Eastern Time.

September Moon Table

Date	Sign	Element	Nature	Phase
1 Tue	Aries	Fire	Barren	3rd
2 Wed 5:02 am	Taurus	Earth	Semi-fruitful	3rd
3 Thu	Taurus	Earth	Semi-fruitful	3rd
4 Fri 7:48 am	Gemini	Air	Barren	3rd
5 Sat	Gemini	Air	Barren	4th 5:54 am
6 Sun 1:40 pm	Cancer	Water	Fruitful	4th
7 Mon	Cancer	Water	Fruitful	4th
8 Tue 10:36 pm	Leo	Fire	Barren	4th
9 Wed	Leo	Fire	Barren	4th
10 Thu	Leo	Fire	Barren	4th
11 Fri 9:56 am	Virgo	Earth	Barren	4th
12 Sat	Virgo	Earth	Barren	4th
13 Sun 10:41 pm	Libra	Air	Semi-fruitful	New 2:41 am
14 Mon	Libra	Air	Semi-fruitful	1st
15 Tue	Libra	Air	Semi-fruitful	1st
16 Wed 11:43 am	Scorpio	Water	Fruitful	1st
17 Thu	Scorpio	Water	Fruitful	1st
18 Fri 11:32 pm	Sagittarius	Fire	Barren	1st
19 Sat	Sagittarius	Fire	Barren	1st
20 Sun	Sagittarius	Fire	Barren	1st
21 Mon 8:33 am	Capricorn	Earth	Semi-fruitful	2nd 4:59 am
22 Tue	Capricorn	Earth	Semi-fruitful	2nd
23 Wed 1:51 pm	Aquarius	Air	Barren	2nd
24 Thu	Aquarius	Air	Barren	2nd
25 Fri 3:43 pm	Pisces	Water	Fruitful	2nd
26 Sat	Pisces	Water	Fruitful	2nd
27 Sun 3:29 pm	Aries	Fire	Barren	Full 10:51 pm
28 Mon	Aries	Fire	Barren	3rd
29 Tue 2:57 pm	Taurus	Earth	Semi-fruitful	3rd
30 Wed	Taurus	Earth	Semi-fruitful	3rd

October Moon Table

Date	Sign	Element	Nature	Phase
1 Thu 4:03 pm	Gemini	Air	Barren	3rd
2 Fri	Gemini	Air	Barren	3rd
3 Sat 8:22 pm	Cancer	Water	Fruitful	3rd
4 Sun	Cancer	Water	Fruitful	4th 5:06 pm
5 Mon	Cancer	Water	Fruitful	4th
6 Tue 4:31 am	Leo	Fire	Barren	4th
7 Wed	Leo	Fire	Barren	4th
8 Thu 3:50 pm	Virgo	Earth	Barren	4th
9 Fri	Virgo	Earth	Barren	4th
10 Sat	Virgo	Earth	Barren	4th
11 Sun 4:45 am	Libra	Air	Semi-fruitful	4th
12 Mon	Libra	Air	Semi-fruitful	New 8:06 pm
13 Tue 5:38 pm	Scorpio	Water	Fruitful	1st
14 Wed	Scorpio	Water	Fruitful	1st
15 Thu	Scorpio	Water	Fruitful	1st
16 Fri 5:18 am	Sagittarius	Fire	Barren	1st
17 Sat	Sagittarius	Fire	Barren	1st
18 Sun 2:52 pm	Capricorn	Earth	Semi-fruitful	1st
19 Mon	Capricorn	Earth	Semi-fruitful	1st
20 Tue 9:38 pm	Aquarius	Air	Barren	2nd 4:31 pm
21 Wed	Aquarius	Air	Barren	2nd
22 Thu	Aquarius	Air	Barren	2nd
23 Fri 1:18 am	Pisces	Water	Fruitful	2nd
24 Sat	Pisces	Water	Fruitful	2nd
25 Sun 2:22 am	Aries	Fire	Barren	2nd
26 Mon	Aries	Fire	Barren	2nd
27 Tue 2:07 am	Taurus	Earth	Semi-fruitful	Full 8:05 am
28 Wed	Taurus	Earth	Semi-fruitful	3rd
29 Thu 2:24 am	Gemini	Air	Barren	3rd
30 Fri	Gemini	Air	Barren	3rd
31 Sat 5:09 am	Cancer	Water	Fruitful	3rd

Times are in Eastern Time.

November Moon Table

Date	Sign	Element	Nature	Phase
1 Sun	Cancer	Water	Fruitful	3rd
2 Mon 10:48 am	Leo	Fire	Barren	3rd
3 Tue	Leo	Fire	Barren	4th 7:24 am
4 Wed 9:22 pm	Virgo	Earth	Barren	4th
5 Thu	Virgo	Earth	Barren	4th
6 Fri	Virgo	Earth	Barren	4th
7 Sat 10:14 am	Libra	Air	Semi-fruitful	4th
8 Sun	Libra	Air	Semi-fruitful	4th
9 Mon 11:02 pm	Scorpio	Water	Fruitful	4th
10 Tue	Scorpio	Water	Fruitful	4th
11 Wed	Scorpio	Water	Fruitful	New 12:47 pm
12 Thu 10:14 am	Sagittarius	Fire	Barren	1st
13 Fri	Sagittarius	Fire	Barren	1st
14 Sat 7:21 pm	Capricorn	Earth	Semi-fruitful	1st
15 Sun	Capricorn	Earth	Semi-fruitful	1st
16 Mon	Capricorn	Earth	Semi-fruitful	1st
17 Tue 2:24 am	Aquarius	Air	Barren	1st
18 Wed	Aquarius	Air	Barren	1st
19 Thu 7:21 am	Pisces	Water	Fruitful	2nd 1:27 am
20 Fri	Pisces	Water	Fruitful	2nd
21 Sat 10:12 am	Aries	Fire	Barren	2nd
22 Sun	Aries	Fire	Barren	2nd
23 Mon 11:26 am	Taurus	Earth	Semi-fruitful	2nd
24 Tue	Taurus	Earth	Semi-fruitful	2nd
25 Wed 12:15 pm	Gemini	Air	Barren	Full 5:44 pm
26 Thu	Gemini	Air	Barren	3rd
27 Fri 2:27 pm	Cancer	Water	Fruitful	3rd
28 Sat	Cancer	Water	Fruitful	3rd
29 Sun 7:47 pm	Leo	Fire	Barren	3rd
30 Mon	Leo	Fire	Barren	3rd

December Moon Table

Date	Sign	Element	Nature	Phase
1 Tue	Leo	Fire	Barren	3rd
2 Wed 5:09 am	Virgo	Earth	Barren	3rd
3 Thu	Virgo	Earth	Barren	4th 2:40 am
4 Fri 5:34 pm	Libra	Air	Semi-fruitful	4th
5 Sat	Libra	Air	Semi-fruitful	4th
6 Sun	Libra	Air	Semi-fruitful	4th
7 Mon 6:26 am	Scorpio	Water	Fruitful	4th
8 Tue	Scorpio	Water	Fruitful	4th
9 Wed 5:25 pm	Sagittarius	Fire	Barren	4th
10 Thu	Sagittarius	Fire	Barren	4th
11 Fri	Sagittarius	Fire	Barren	New 5:29 am
12 Sat 1:46 am	Capricorn	Earth	Semi-fruitful	1st
13 Sun	Capricorn	Earth	Semi-fruitful	1st
14 Mon 7:59 am	Aquarius	Air	Barren	1st
15 Tue	Aquarius	Air	Barren	1st
16 Wed 12:45 pm	Pisces	Water	Fruitful	1st
17 Thu	Pisces	Water	Fruitful	1st
18 Fri 4:26 pm	Aries	Fire	Barren	2nd 10:14 am
19 Sat	Aries	Fire	Barren	2nd
20 Sun 7:13 pm	Taurus	Earth	Semi-fruitful	2nd
21 Mon	Taurus	Earth	Semi-fruitful	2nd
22 Tue 9:31 pm	Gemini	Air	Barren	2nd
23 Wed	Gemini	Air	Barren	2nd
24 Thu	Gemini	Air	Barren	2nd
25 Fri 12:27 am	Cancer	Water	Fruitful	Full 6:12 am
26 Sat	Cancer	Water	Fruitful	3rd
27 Sun 5:31 am	Leo	Fire	Barren	3rd
28 Mon	Leo	Fire	Barren	3rd
29 Tue 1:58 pm	Virgo	Earth	Barren	3rd
30 Wed	Virgo	Earth	Barren	3rd
31 Thu	Virgo	Eart	Barren	3rd

Times are in Eastern Time.

Dates to Destroy Weeds and Pests

Dates	Sign	Quarter
Jan 6, 6:03 am–Jan 8, 5:58 pm	Leo	3rd
Jan 8, 5:58 pm–Jan 11, 6:57 am	Virgo	3rd
Jan 16, 3:01 am–Jan 18, 7:04 am	Sagittarius	4th
Jan 20, 7:59 am–Jan 20, 8:14 am	Aquarius	4th
Feb 3, 6:09 pm–Feb 5, 12:46 am	Leo	3rd
Feb 5, 12:46 am–Feb 7, 1:44 pm	Virgo	3rd
Feb 12, 11:46 am–Feb 14, 5:24 pm	Sagittarius	4th
Feb 16, 7:13 pm–Feb 18, 6:47 pm	Aquarius	4th
Mar 5, 1:05 pm–Mar 6, 7:52 pm	Virgo	3rd
Mar 11, 7:30 pm–Mar 13, 1:48 pm	Sagittarius	3rd
Mar 13, 1:48 pm–Mar 14, 2:40 am	Sagittarius	4th
Mar 16, 6:14 am–Mar 18, 6:58 am	Aquarius	4th
Apr 8, 1:08 am–Apr 10, 8:47 am	Sagittarius	3rd
Apr 12, 1:44 pm–Apr 14, 4:12 pm	Aquarius	4th
Apr 16, 5:00 pm–Apr 18, 2:57 pm	Aries	4th
May 5, 7:13 am–May 7, 2:16 pm	Sagittarius	3rd
May 9, 7:22 pm–May 11, 6:36 am	Aquarius	3rd
May 11, 6:36 am–May 11, 10:53 pm	Aquarius	4th
May 14, 1:13 am–May 16, 3:02 am	Aries	4th
Jun 2, 12:19 pm–Jun 3, 8:50 pm	Sagittarius	3rd
Jun 6, 1:02 am–Jun 8, 4:16 am	Aquarius	3rd
Jun 10, 7:14 am–Jun 12, 10:16 am	Aries	4th
Jun 14, 1:51 pm–Jun 16, 10:05 am	Gemini	4th
Jul 3, 8:21 am–Jul 5, 10:23 am	Aquarius	3rd
Jul 7, 12:38 pm–Jul 8, 4:24 pm	Aries	3rd

Dates to Destroy Weeds and Pests

Dates	Sign	Quarter
Jul 8, 4:24 pm–Jul 9, 3:49 pm	Aries	4th
Jul 11, 8:16 pm–Jul 14, 2:14 am	Gemini	4th
Jul 31, 6:43 am–Aug 1, 6:36 pm	Aquarius	3rd
Aug 3, 7:24 pm–Aug 5, 9:29 pm	Aries	3rd
Aug 8, 1:40 am–Aug 10, 8:08 am	Gemini	4th
Aug 12, 4:52 pm–Aug 14, 10:53 am	Leo	4th
Aug 31, 4:33 am–Sep 2, 5:02 am	Aries	3rd
Sep 4, 7:48 am–Sep 5, 5:54 am	Gemini	3rd
Sep 5, 5:54 am–Sep 6, 1:40 pm	Gemini	4th
Sep 8, 10:36 pm–Sep 11, 9:56 am	Leo	4th
Sep 11, 9:56 am–Sep 13, 2:41 am	Virgo	4th
Sep 27, 10:51 pm–Sep 29, 2:57 pm	Aries	3rd
Oct 1, 4:03 pm–Oct 3, 8:22 pm	Gemini	3rd
Oct 6, 4:31 am–Oct 8, 3:50 pm	Leo	4th
Oct 8, 3:50 pm–Oct 11, 4:45 am	Virgo	4th
Oct 29, 2:24 am–Oct 31, 5:09 am	Gemini	3rd
Nov 2, 10:48 am–Nov 3, 7:24 am	Leo	3rd
Nov 3, 7:24 am–Nov 4, 9:22 pm	Leo	4th
Nov 4, 9:22 pm–Nov 7, 10:14 am	Virgo	4th
Nov 25, 5:44 pm–Nov 27, 2:27 pm	Gemini	3rd
Nov 29, 7:47 pm–Dec 2, 5:09 am	Leo	3rd
Dec 2, 5:09 am–Dec 3, 2:40 am	Virgo	3rd
Dec 3, 2:40 am–Dec 4, 5:34 pm	Virgo	4th
Dec 9, 5:25 pm–Dec 11, 5:29 am	Sagittarius	4th
Dec 27, 5:31 am–Dec 29, 1:58 pm	Leo	3rd

Times are in Eastern Time.

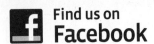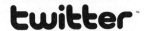
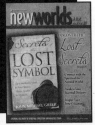